Hodgkin Lymphoma

Editors

VOLKER DIEHL
PETER BORCHMANN

HEMATOLOGY/ONCOLOGY CLINICS OF NORTH AMERICA

www.hemonc.theclinics.com

Consulting Editors
GEORGE P. CANELLOS
H. FRANKLIN BUNN

February 2014 • Volume 28 • Number 1

ELSEVIER

1600 John F. Kennedy Boulevard • Suite 1800 • Philadelphia, Pennsylvania, 19103-2899

http://www.theclinics.com

HEMATOLOGY/ONCOLOGY CLINICS OF NORTH AMERICA Volume 28, Number 1
February 2014 ISSN 0889-8588, ISBN 13: 978-0-323-26660-4

Editor: Jessica McCool
Developmental Editor: Donald Mumford

Hematology/Oncology Clinics (ISSN 0889-8588) is published bimonthly by Elsevier Inc., 360 Park Avenue South, New York, NY 10010-1710. Months of issue are February, April, June, August, October, and December. Business and Editorial Offices: 1600 John F. Kennedy Blvd., Ste. 1800, Philadelphia, PA 19103–2899. Customer Service Office: 3251 Riverport Lane, Maryland Heights, MO63043. Periodicals postage paid at New York, NY and at additional mailing offices. Subscription prices are $385.00 per year (domestic individuals), $633.00 per year (domestic institutions), $190.00 per year (domestic students/residents), $440.00 per year (Canadian individuals), $783.00 per year (Canadian institutions) $520.00 per year (international individuals), $783.00 per year (international institutions), and $255.00 per year (international and Canadian students/residents). International air speed delivery is included in all Clinics subscription prices. All prices are subject to change without notice. **POSTMASTER:** Send address changes to Hematology/Oncology Clinics of North America, Elsevier Health Sciences Division, Subscription Customer Service, 3251 Riverport Lane, Maryland Heights, MO 63043. Customer Service (orders, claims, online, change of address): Elsevier Health Sciences Division, Subscription Customer Service, 3251 Riverport Lane, Maryland Heights, MO 63043. Tel: 1-800-654-2452 (U.S. and Canada); 314-447-8871 (outside U.S. and Canada). Fax: 314-447-8029. E-mail: journalscustomerservice-usa@elsevier.com (for print support); journalsonlinesupport-usa@elsevier.com (for online support).

Reprints. For copies of 100 or more, of articles in this publication, please contact the Commercial Reprints Department, Elsevier Inc., 360 Park Avenue South, New York, New York 10010-1710; Tel.: 212-633-3874, Fax: 212-633-3820, E-mail: reprints@elsevier.com.

Hematology/Oncology Clinics of North America is covered in MEDLINE/PubMed (Index Medicus), EMBASE/ Excerpta Medica, and BIOSIS.

Printed and bound by CPI Group (UK) Ltd, Croydon, CR0 4YY

Transferred to digital print 2012

Contributors

CONSULTING EDITORS

GEORGE P. CANELLOS, MD
William Rosenberg Professor of Medicine, Department of Medical Oncology, Dana-Farber Cancer Institute, Boston, Massachusetts

H. FRANKLIN BUNN, MD
Professor of Medicine, Division of Hematology, Brigham and Women's Hospital, Harvard Medical School, Boston, Massachusetts

EDITORS

VOLKER DIEHL, MD, PhD
Professor of Medicine, Emeritus, Director, 1st Department of Internal Medicine, University of Cologne, Cologne, Germany

PETER BORCHMANN, MD, PhD
Professor, 1st Department of Internal Medicine, German Hodgkin Study Group, University Hospital Cologne, Cologne, Germany

AUTHORS

RANJANA ADVANI, MD
Professor of Medicine, Medicine/Oncology, Stanford University Medical Center, Stanford, California

STEPHEN C. ALLEY, PhD
Seattle Genetics Inc, Bothell, Washington

MARC P.E. ANDRÉ, MD
Professor of Hematology, CHU Dinant Godinne, UCL Namur, Yvoir, Belgium

STEPHEN M. ANSELL, MD, PhD
Professor of Medicine, Division of Hematology, Mayo Clinic, Rochester, Minnesota

PETER BORCHMANN, MD, PhD
Professor, 1st Department of Internal Medicine, German Hodgkin Study Group, University Hospital Cologne, Cologne, Germany

CATHERINE DIEFENBACH, MD
Assistant Professor of Medicine, Department of Medicine, New York University School of Medicine, New York University Cancer Center, New York, New York

VOLKER DIEHL, MD, PhD
Professor of Medicine, Emeritus, Director, 1st Department of Internal Medicine, University of Cologne, Cologne, Germany

ANNETTE E. HAY, MB ChB, MRCP, FRCPath
Clinical Fellow, NCIC Clinical Trials Group, Queen's University, Kingston, Ontario, Canada

MARK HERTZBERG, MBBS, PhD, FRACP, FRCPA
Professor, Department of Haematology, Westmead Hospital, Westmead,
New South Wales, Australia

MARTIN HUTCHINGS, MD, PhD
Staff Specialist, Department of Haematology, Rigshospitalet, Copenhagen, Denmark

RALPH M. MEYER, MD, FRCP(C)
President, Juravinski Hospital and Cancer Centre, Regional Vice President, Cancer Care
Ontario, Hamilton, Ontario, Canada

NICOLE M. OKELEY, PhD
Seattle Genetics Inc, Bothell, Washington

PETER D. SENTER, PhD
Seattle Genetics Inc, Bothell, Washington

HARALD STEIN, MD, PhD
Professor of Pathology, Emeritus, Former Director, Institute for Pathology, Campus
Benjamin Franklin, Charité University Medicine Berlin; Chairman, Berlin Reference and
Consultation Center for Lymphoma and Hematopathology, Pathodiagnostik Berlin, Berlin,
Germany

ANAS YOUNES, MD
Lymphoma Service, Memorial Sloan-Kettering Cancer Center, New York, New York

Contents

> Hodgkin's disease (HD) is a fatal disorder with the unique histologic fea-
> tures of few dysplastic Hodgkin- and Reed-Sternberg (HRS) cells sur-
> rounded by an abundance of nonatypical bystander cells in primary
> biopsies. By using the first Hodgkin cell line L428 the cytokine receptor
> CD30 was discovered. CD30 proved to be an excellent target for the diag-
> noses of CD30+ malignancies and for monoclonal antibody therapy in
> patients with these malignancies because of its highly restricted expression
> in healthy individuals. Recently, a new anti-CD30-toxin-drug-conjugate
> consisting of an anti-CD30 monoclonal antibody bound to the nonimmuno-
> genic toxin auristatin E with a newly designed linker was generated.

> The concept of using monoclonal antibodies for delivering drugs to cancer
> cells has been explored for decades, with early work surrounding nonspe-
> cific targets and drugs with low potencies. These studies underscored the
> importance of critical parameters, such as antigen and tumor target selec-
> tion, linker stability, drug potency, pharmacokinetics, and conjugation meth-
> odology, in developing effective antibody drug conjugates with acceptable
> safety profiles. Brentuximab vedotin represents the culmination of much
> research and development activities in which many of these parameters
> were addressed. This article provides an overview of many studies that
> led to the development of this highly active antibody drug conjugate.

> Hodgkin lymphoma (HL) is a relatively rare but highly curable human can-
> cer. Because very few patients relapse and will require subsequent ther-
> apy, new drug development for HL has not been seen as a high priority
> by the pharmaceutical industry. Brentuximab vedotin, an antibody-drug
> conjugate that targets CD30 receptors, became the first drug to be
> approved by regulatory agencies for the treatment of HL in more than 30
> years. This review summarizes the current and future directions of incorpo-
> rating brentuximab vedotin in the management of patients with HL.

> Combination chemoradiotherapy achieves excellent results for the treat-
> ment of localized Hodgkin lymphoma. However, late toxic effects occur,

mostly related to the radiotherapy administered after the standard adria-mycin, bleomycin, vinblastine, and dacarbazine (ABVD) chemotherapy. The most serious sequelae are radiation-induced secondary cancers. Reducing radiotherapy has not yet prevented late malignancies. However, when radiotherapy was omitted, tumor control was inferior, with more relapses necessitating rescue treatment including high-dose chemother-apy with stem cell support. Early fluorodeoxyglucose positron emission tomography performed after a few cycles of ABVD is evaluated in several randomized trials to identify patients who might be safely treated with che-motherapy alone.

Because long-term survival of patients with nonbulky stage IA to IIA Hodg-kin lymphoma is dependent on disease control and avoidance of late toxic effects associated with the treatment received, the initial choice of treat-ment can be associated with trade-offs that balance optimum disease control with avoidance of these late effect risks. Health professionals and patients face the dilemma of making treatment decisions without the benefit of completely understanding the risk-benefit balances associ-ated with how current treatments affect all outcomes of interest. Optimum management of these patients requires careful multidisciplinary evaluation and communication strategies that account for patient preferences.

The key question in advanced-stage Hodgkin lymphoma for many years now has been, should intensified chemotherapy be applied upfront or be reserved for relapsing patients. The early intensification approach with BEACOPP$_{escalated}$ (bleomycin, etoposide, doxorubicin, cyclophospha-mide, vincristine, procarbazine, prednisone) aims at curing patients with first-line chemotherapy definitely. The added toxicity of this approach as compared to less intensive regimens as ABDV (doxorubicin, bleomycin, dacarbazine, vinblastine) is mainly restricted to acute haematotoxicity and gonadal damage. However, regarding efficacy, there is a meaningful survival-benefit over ABVD (10% at 5 years) and the intensified first-line treatment strategy is thus rightly regarded as standard of care.

The goal of therapy for patients with advanced-stage Hodgkin lymphoma is to ensure that as many patients as possible are healthy and free of dis-ease decades after completing treatment. To achieve this, the treating physician needs to select the most effective therapeutic regimen, but also needs to choose a treatment strategy that limits long-term toxicity. One approach to achieve this is to use a less intense combination, such as ABVD chemotherapy, as initial treatment and intensify therapy only in those patients who do not become PET negative or who subsequently relapse.

Fluorodeoxyglucose (FDG) positron emission tomography (PET)/computed tomography (CT) is the most accurate tool for staging, treatment monitoring, and response evaluation in Hodgkin lymphoma (HL). Early determination of treatment sensitivity by FDG-PET is the best tool to guide individualized, response-adapted treatment. Several ongoing or recently completed trials have investigated the use of FDG-PET/CT for early response-adapted HL therapy. The results are encouraging, but the data are immature, and PET response–adapted HL therapy is discouraged outside the setting of clinical trials. PET/CT looks promising for selection of therapy in relapsed and refractory disease, but the role in this setting is still unclear.

Although most patients with Hodgkin lymphoma (HL) are cured with primary therapy, patients with primary refractory disease or relapse after initial treatment have poor outcomes and represent an unmet medical need. Recent advances in unraveling the biology of HL have yielded a plethora of novel targeted therapies. This review provides an overview of the data behind the hype generated by these advances and addresses the question of whether or not clinically these targeted therapies offer hope for patients with HL.

For relapsed-refractory Hodgkin Lymphoma, standard therapy consists of salvage chemotherapy followed by autologous stem cell transplantation. Adverse risk factors at relapse include response duration less than 12 months, advanced stage, extranodal disease, "B" symptoms and anemia. There is no obvious superior salvage regimen although maintaining dose-intensity is important for optimal responses. Assessment of response to salvage using FDG-PET identifies a distinct poor risk group, especially those with extranodal disease. Either a second salvage regimen or a tandem autologous transplant may benefit some patients with residual disease post-salvage. Reduced-intensity allografting may provide durable responses for some patients relapsing post-autologous transplant.

HEMATOLOGY/ONCOLOGY CLINICS OF NORTH AMERICA

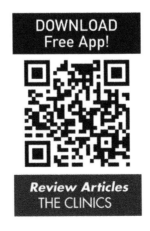

DOWNLOAD
Free App!

Review Articles
THE CLINICS

NOW AVAILABLE FOR YOUR iPhone and iPad

Preface

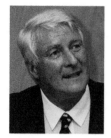 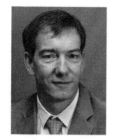

Volker Diehl, MD, PhD   Peter Borchmann, MD, PhD
Editors

As early as in 1666, Marcello Malpighi described in his script, "De Viscerum Structuru Exercitatio Anatomica," a clinical syndrome of enlarged lymph nodes and a large spleen, a clinical phenomenon that was again meticulously described in1832 by Thomas Hodgkin in his publication, "On Some Morbid Appearances of the Absorbent Glands and Spleen," in the *Medico-Chirurgical Transactions* in London. When Samuel Wilks made similar observations in 1865, he was generous enough to give credit to Thomas Hodgkin and called this clinical syndrome for the first time "Hodgkin's disease." In 1994 Hodgkin disease became "Hodgkin lymphoma" (HL) when Ralph Küppers in our group in Cologne resolved the 160-year-old puzzle: is Hodgkin disease an infection, an inflammation, or a true malignant lymphoma? Ralph Küppers discovered that the pathognomonic "Hodgkin/Reed-Sternberg cells" (HRS cells) are bona fide malignant monoclonal B lymphocytes designating Hodgkin disease a true cancer!

HL is a unique cancer characterized by the exceptional histology with a minority of tumor cells embraced by a plethora of nutritive bystander cells, making this mediator-driven scenario a classic example of microenvironment-tumor cell interaction. Furthermore, the high chemo-radiosensitivity of the HRS cells, the young age of the patients, and the over 90% curability of all stages of the disease make this lymphoma entity a stand-alone in adulthood cancers.

In this issue, the reader will learn about the onset of modern cell biology, resulting in the first HRS-cell line ever cultured in vitro, which gave rise to the molecular insights of the lymphomagenesis of HL. With the detection of the CD30 antigen on the HRS cells in culture opened an unprecedented change of therapeutic possibilities. A "magic bullet" could be constructed; an antibody-drug-conjugate (ADC) called brentuximab vedotin, whereby a linker-bound cytostatic MMAE (aurostatin) is targeted via the anti-CD30 antibody to the HRS cell. It is then engulfed and exerts its antimitotic activity, resulting in cell death of the HRS cells followed by the collapse of the microenvironment. The first clinical proofs of the high tumor reductive potential of brentuximab vedotin in US phase I-II trials are reported in this issue.

Despite the enormous treatment successes in all strata of the disease, there are pending controversies how to best treat patients in the different stages. These controversies are carefully addressed in this issue. Should we give chemo-radiotherapy

Hematol Oncol Clin N Am 28 (2014) ix–x
http://dx.doi.org/10.1016/j.hoc.2013.10.011
0889-8588/14/$ – see front matter © 2014 Elsevier Inc. All rights reserved.

in early stages or do we cure patients in localized stages with chemotherapy alone? What is the right first-line treatment in disseminated stages of HL, the North American dogma, starting with ABVD and—as late intensification strategy—necessitating 35% salvage therapy with high-dose therapy followed by hematopoietic stem cell support? Or should we use escalated BEACOPP as early intensification—the European strategy—leading to a 20% better tumor response but accompanied by a significant higher acute toxicity and necessitating only in 5% to 10% salvage therapy?

Finally, the enormous plethora of new molecules interfering with aberrant intracellular pathways and antibodies or ADCs directed against surface markers on the tumor cells are described and put in scene for the improvement of options and better outcome of patients with relapsing and refractory HL.

Volker Diehl, MD, PhD
1st Department of Internal Medicine, University of Cologne
Joseph Stelzmannstrasse
Cologne 50937, Germany

Peter Borchmann, MD, PhD
1st Department of Internal Medicine
German Hodgkin Study Group
University Hospital Cologne
Kerpener Straße 62
Cologne 50924, Germany

E-mail addresses:
v.diehl@uni-koeln.de (V. Diehl)
peter.borchmann@uni-koeln.de (P. Borchmann)

First Hodgkin Cell Line L428 and the CD30 Antigen
Their Role for Diagnostic and Treatment of CD30-positive Neoplasms

Harald Stein, MD, PhD[a], Volker Diehl, MD, PhD[b],*

KEYWORDS

- Hodgkin lymphoma • Establishment of the cell line L428
- Detection of the CD30 Antigen

KEY POINTS

- Hodgkin's disease (HD) is a fatal disorder with the unique histologic features of few dysplastic Hodgkin- and Reed-Sternberg (HRS) cells surrounded by an abundance of nonatypical bystander cells in primary biopsies.
- By using the first Hodgkin cell line L428 the cytokine receptor CD30 was discovered.
- CD30 proved to be an excellent target for the diagnoses of CD30+ malignancies and for monoclonal antibody therapy in patients with these malignancies because of its highly restricted expression in healthy individuals.
- Recently, a new anti-CD30-toxin-drug-conjugate consisting of an anti-CD30 monoclonal antibody bound to the nonimmunogenic toxin auristatin E with a newly designed linker was generated.

WHY WAS IT ESSENTIAL TO ESTABLISH A HODGKIN CELL LINE?

When the histology of Hodgkin disease (HD) was investigated (1898 first by Sternberg[1] and 4 years later by Reed[2]), an unusual cellular composition for a fatal disorder was observed (**Fig. 1**). Most of the cells in the affected lymph nodes proved to be nonatypical bystander cells (ie, lymphocytes, plasma cells, histiocytes, neutrophilic and/or eosinophilic granulocytes, and others). The atypical large mononuclear and multinuclear blastoid cells, called Hodgkin and Reed-Sternberg (HRS) cells, were found in the minority, ranging from 0.1% to 1% of all cells present in the specimen.[3] Because of this, it was thought that HD is more likely an infectious disease or an inflammatory

[a] Berlin Reference and Consultation Center for Lymphoma and Hematopathology, Pathodiagnostik Berlin, Komturstrasse 58-62, Berlin 12099, Germany; [b] Clinic I for Internal Medicine, University of Cologne, 50937 Köln, Joseph Stelzmannstr, Germany
* Corresponding author.
E-mail address: v.diehl@uni-koeln.de

Hematol Oncol Clin N Am 28 (2014) 1–11
http://dx.doi.org/10.1016/j.hoc.2013.10.007
0889-8588/14/$ – see front matter © 2014 Elsevier Inc. All rights reserved.

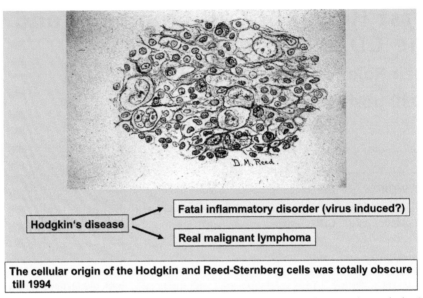

Fig. 1. There were 2 concepts about the nature of HD. (*From* Reed D. On the pathological changes in Hodgkin's disease, with special reference to its relation to tuberculosis. Johns Hopkins Hosp Rep 1902;10:133–96.)

process than a true neoplasm. The rarity of the HRS cells and the abundance of surrounding bystander cells made the investigation of HRS cells with special techniques impossible.

THE ESTABLISHMENT OF THE L428 CELL LINE

To obtain pure HRS cells in large quantities, many laboratories tried to establish long-term in vitro cultures of primary HRS cells when in the 1960s and 1970s suitable culture conditions like RPMI media together with fetal calf serum became available. All attempts by Zech and colleagues,[4] Kaplan and Gartner,[5] and many others were unsuccessful. The same was true for the 427 culture attempts by Volker Diehl and his group between 1969 and 1978 at the Radiumhemmet/Karolinska Sjukhuset in Stockholm/Sweden and later in Hannover/Germany. Most of the culture attempts resulted in Epstein-Barr virus-transformed lymphoblastoid cell cultures. After his relocation to Hannover, Diehl continued with the attempts to establish in vitro cultures of Hodgkin-Reed-Sternberg cells and succeeded with his team in 1979 in growing for the first time a permanently growing Epstein-Barr virus-negative cell line from a pleural effusion of a young female patient with nodular sclerosing HD (**Table 1**).[6,7]

Features of the L428 Hodgkin Cell Line

This cell line was designated L428, because it was the 428th culture attempt. The in vitro proliferating cells proved to be aneuploid, carrying several marker chromosomes (1p+, 2p+, 6q+, 7q+, 9p+, 11q−, 13p+, 21q−). The total number of chromosomes per cell amounted to 48–50.[7] These findings demonstrated that the L428 cell-line cells were monoclonal and derived from a very atypical cell population. Immunophenotypical studies revealed an absence of B-cell-, T-cell-, and macrophage markers (**Fig. 2**A).[7] Considering these findings, it was tempting to assume that the

Table 1
Clinical data of patient E.M. from whom L-428 cells were established

Year	Histology	Stage	Therapy	Result
2/1972	Nod. sclerosis	II, B supracl. LN, mediast. LN	Ext. RT	CR
2/1974	Relapse, NS	IVE, B, chest wall infiltration, pleural effusion	Chemo-radiotherapy: COPP-ABVD+ RT	PR → Progressive disease
11/1974	Progression	→	Palliation Pleural tappings 2–4 wk before death[a]	Death

[a] Time points of pleural tappings for in vitro cell cultures.

L428 cells were direct derivatives from HRS cells. In addition, the disease report of the donor patient (see **Table 1**) of the L428 cell line supported this conclusion.

Despite the mentioned findings and especially because of the disappointing publications by Kaplan and Gartner[5] and Long and colleagues,[8] there was general hesitation in the scientific community to accept the L428 cell line as a true Hodgkin cell line.[9] In this situation Diehl approached Stein with the request to establish arguments that could help to show that the L428 cell line cells were real derivatives from in vivo HRS cells.

What Stein did first was to incubate the L428 cells with his own T cells. This experiment showed that the L428 cells bind T cells in rosette formation like primary HRS cells (Stein H, unpublished observation, 1980) (see **Fig. 2**C) and was an important further criterion for the assumption that the L428 cells represent true HRS cells.

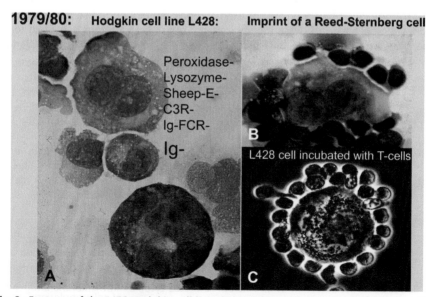

Fig. 2. Features of the L428 Hodgkin cell line. (*From* Schaadt M, Diehl V, Stein H, et al. Two neoplastic cell lines with unique features derived from Hodgkin's disease. Int J Cancer 1980;26(6):723–31; with permission.)

DISCOVERY OF THE CD30 ANTIGEN AND ITS APPLICATION IN RESEARCH, DIAGNOSTIC, AND THERAPY
Detection of HRS-cell-related Antigens by Rabbit Polyclonal Antisera

To detect HRS-cell-specific antigens, Stein's team immunized rabbits with the L428 cell-line cells. Two rabbit antisera selectively immunostained HRS cells following absorption with neutrophils and Daudi-cell-line cells. One antiserum stained the nuclei and the other antiserum stained the cytoplasm of HRS cells (**Fig. 3**).[10,11]

Detection of the Proliferation-Associated Antigen Ki-67 and the HRS-cell-Related Antigen Ki-1

Ki-1 by the monoclonal antibody approach
To generate a permanent source of antibodies that react selectively with HRS cells, the L428 cells were subjected to the monoclonal antibody (moab) approach. More than 3000 hybridoma supernatants were screened by immunostaining frozen sections of a Hodgkin case, a tonsil, and L428 cells. Two monoclonal antibodies reactive with HRS cells could be identified. One moab called Ki-67 did not only react with the nuclei of HRS cells but also reacted with the nuclei of germinal center cells.[12] Further studies confirmed that Ki-67 is a proliferation-associated antigen that is expressed throughout the whole cell cycle but not in resting cells.[13] The other moab, called Ki-1, confirmed the existence of an antigen that is highly restricted to HRS cells and is present on the surface membrane and the cytoplasm of HRS cells (**Fig. 4**A).[14,15] In normal lymphoid tissues the Ki-1 antigen was encountered only on a few mononuclear blastoid cells usually located in the perifollicular area of secondary follicles (**Fig. 4**B).

CD30 as a Diagnostic Target: Identification of a New Lymphoma Entity and Its Detection in Formol-fixed and Paraffin-embedded Tissue Sections

With the aid of the Ki-1 antibody, Stein and colleagues[16,17] detected a new lymphoma disease, which they designated *anaplastic large cell lymphoma (ALCL)*. Because the Ki-1 antibody did not work on formol-fixed and paraffin-embedded sections, a broad diagnostic application of this antibody was not possible. Therefore, the Stein team generated new monoclonal antibodies to the Ki-1 antigen. Among the 10 new

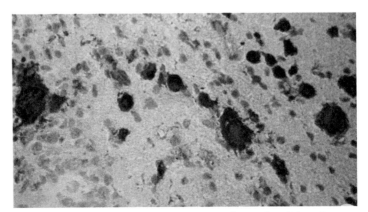

Fig. 3. 1980/01: First detection of an HRS-cell restricted cytoplasmic/membrane antigen by immunostaining of a frozen section from a classical Hodgkin lymphoma with a rabbit polyclonal antiserum raised against the L428 cell line and absorbed with neutrophils and Daudi cell line cells.

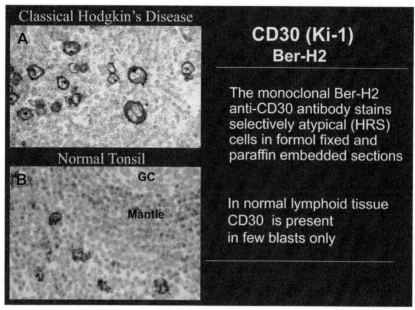

Fig. 4. Selective immunostaining of CD30 cells in formol-fixed and paraffin-embedded tissue section from classical HD and human tonsils with the monoclonal anti-CD30 antibody Ber-H2. GC, germinal center.

monoclonal antibodies directed to the Ki-1 antigen, there was one, designated BerH2, which selectively and reliably immunostained HRS cells in routinely formol-fixed and in paraffin-embedded tissue sections (see **Fig. 4**A).[18] Thanks to the availability of Ber-H2 and further anti-Ki-1 antibodies, the monoclonal anti-Ki-1 antibodies were clustered at the Leukocyte Typing workshop at Oxford in 1986 and received the cluster designation CD30.[19] With the availability of the monoclonal anti-CD30 Ber-H2, CD30 became the most important marker for CD30-associated diseases with special reference to HD and ALCL. The broad screening of normal tissues confirmed the highly restricted expression of CD30 in healthy individuals. Labeling of biopsies from patients with classical Hodgkin lymphoma (CHL) for CD30 revealed that HRS cells exhibit a greater morphologic variability as previously known and are often much more frequent, ranging up to 30% of the cells in the affected tissue (**Fig. 5**). All nuclei in the multinucleated RS cells are Ki-67 positive, indicating that all the nuclei present in these multinucleated cells take part in the proliferation process (insert in **Fig. 5**).

Biosynthesis and Structure of CD30 and Shedding as a Soluble Form

The CD30 molecule is synthesized as a 90-kDa precursor protein, which is expressed as a 120-kDa at the surface membrane.[20] It can be shed in a soluble form.[21] The measurement of its level in the serum can be used to monitor the disease activity of CHL and ALCL.[22] Molecular cloning of the CD30 gene revealed in 1992 that the CD30 protein is a cytokine receptor of the tumor necrosis factor receptor family.[23] Structurally, CD30 proved to be a type 1 transmembrane protein that contains 6 cysteine-rich repeat motifs in its extracellular domain. The cytoplasmic tail contains several tumor necrosis factor receptor-associated factor–binding sequences that can mediate activation of the nuclear factor kB (**Fig. 6**). The CD30 gene has been assigned to chromosome 1p36.[24]

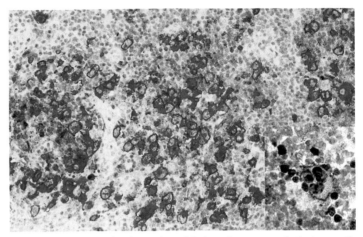

Fig. 5. CD30 immunostaining of a classical Hodkin lymphoma reveals that more than 30% of the cells present in the affected tissue can be HRS cells and demonstrates that HRS cells can be much more frequent than assumed before the availability of anti-CD30 antibodies. The double labeling for CD30 in red and Ki-67 in black (insert) shows that HRS cells are Ki-67-positive and thus in proliferation and not silent.

Derivation and Molecular Characteristics of HRS Cells

The cellular origin and nature of HRS cells were an enigma since their first description. Moab to CD30 enabled the isolation of single HRS cells from frozen sections (**Fig. 7**) and their investigation by a single-cell PCR assay (see **Fig. 7**). In 1994 and the following years, this approach led to the finding that HRS cells represent disabled monoclonal and thus neoplastic B cells since they consistently harbour monoclonal immunoglobulin (IG) rearrangements. The HRS cells are disabled because of a defect

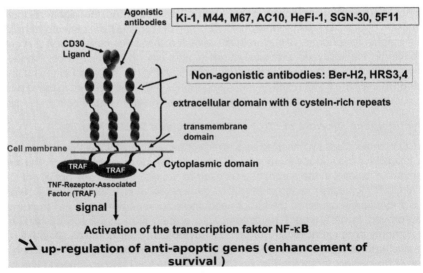

Fig. 6. Molecular structure and function of CD30.

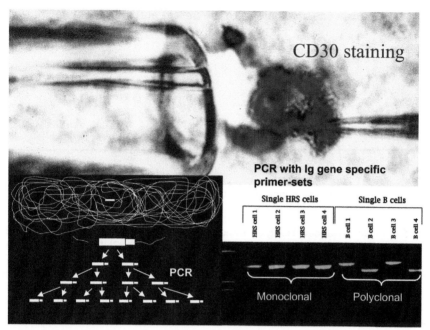

Fig. 7. Picking and isolation of a single CD30-positive HRS cell from a frozen classical Hodgkin lymphoma section and the result of the PCR with IG gene-specific primer sets of picked single CD30 HRS cells in comparison of picked bystander single B cells.

in IG transcription. This is not due to crippled rearranged IG genes[25] since 75% of the rearranged IG genes are functional but because of a lack of the transcription factors Oct2a and BOB.1.[26] These findings induced the editorial team of the World Health Organization lymphoma classification to change the term Hodgkin's disease into classical Hodgkin lymphoma.[3]

Hodgkin Lymphoma Includes 2 Different Entities

Investigations using CD30 and CD20 as cell markers confirmed that HD is composed of 2 different lymphoma disease entities: one is the CD20+ CD30− nodular lymphocyte-predominant HL and the other the CD30+ CD20− CHL.

CD30 as a Therapeutic Target

Studies with naked anti-CD30 antibodies and the first anti-CD30-drug conjugate
CD30 is an excellent target for moab therapy in patients with CD30+ malignancies because of its highly restricted expression in healthy individuals. Therefore, many times it was attempted to target CD30+ lymphoma cells with naked anti-CD30 antibodies.[27–29] Significant responses were not observed. Therefore for the first time in 1992 the anti-CD30 antibody was conjugated to a toxin, which was saporin, a potent single-chain ribosome-inactivating protein from *Saponaria officinalis* (**Fig. 8**).[30] With this conjugate a rapid but only transient tumor reduction was achieved in 3 of 4 patients with advanced CHL (**Fig. 9**). The administration of the conjugate could not be repeated because the patients developed high antibody titers to both parts of the conjugate. Notwithstanding this problem, this result of an antibody-mediated tumor

The toxin saporin is linked to the Ber-H2 anti-CD30 antibody

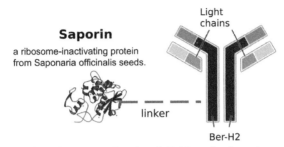

Fig. 8. Structure of the first monoclonal anti-CD30 antibody-toxin conjugate.

reduction of an advanced Hodgkin tumor represented, to the best of the authors' knowledge, the first proof of principle of targeted therapy in CHL. Another important finding of this study was that the anti-CD30–saporin-conjugate injected into the patient intravenously found its way to the HRS cells despite the presence of a very strong fibrotic tissue of nodular sclerosing HL after the preceding radiotherapy and chemotherapy, which was demonstrated by the fact that the HRS cells could be immunostained with an antimurine IgG antibody on a biopsy taken 24 hours following intravenous injection of the Ber-H2-saporin conjugate.

Breakthrough in CD30-targeted antibody therapy
It took more than 20 years until the potent nonimmunogenic toxin auristatin E was developed from the Indian Ocean sera hare, *Dolabela auricularia*.[31] Auristatin E exerts its toxin activity through inhibiting tubulin polymerization. A further important step was the development of a special linker (valin-citrulline dipeptide) by which the auristatin E is conjugated to the anti-CD30 antibody (**Fig. 10**).[31,32] The binding by this linker provides good stability of the conjugate in the plasma. As long as the auristatin E is linked

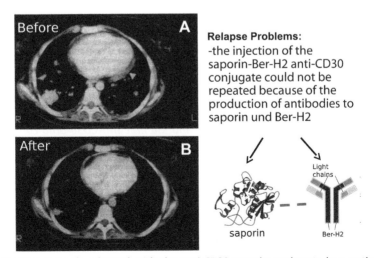

Fig. 9. Treatment result achieved with the anti-CD30-saporin conjugate in a patient with classical Hodgkin lymphoma.

Breakthrough in the CD30 target antibody therapy
by a conjugate consisting of a monoclonal anti-CD30 antibody, a cleavable linker, a spacer and the non-immunogenic toxin auristation E.

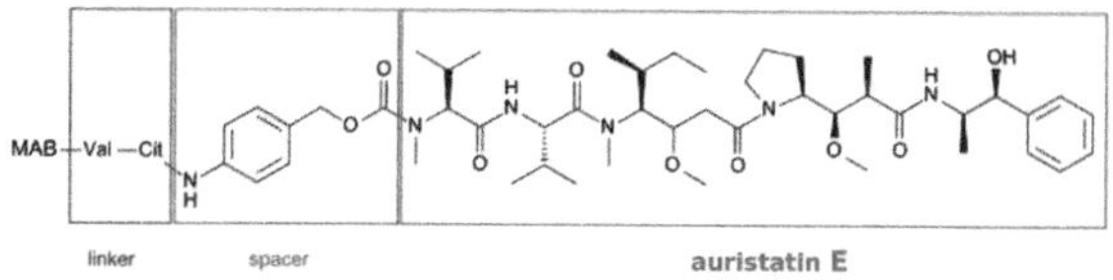

linker   spacer   auristatin E

Mechanism of action
Auristatin E is an anti-mitotic agent which inhibits cell division by blocking polymerization of tubulin. The valine-citrulline dipeptide which links auristatin E to the monoclonal anti-CD30 antibody is stable in extracellular fluid, but is cleaved by cathepsin once the conjugate has entered a CD30+ tumor cell. The released auristatin E exerts its antimitotic action by which the tumor cell is killed.

Fig. 10. Breakthrough in the CD30 targeted antibody therapy. (*From* Doronina SO, Toki BE, Torgov MY, et al. Development of potent monoclonal antibody auristatin conjugates for cancer therapy. Nat Biotechnol 2003;21(7):778–84; with permission.)

to the anti-CD30 antibody, it is not toxic. When the anti-CD30 antibody-auristatin conjugate has reached the target cell and is internalized, auristatin E is released from the antibody and becomes toxic and kills the cell. There is evidence that not only is the targeted CD30-positive cell killed, but also CD30-negative cells in the neighborhood.[33] The presumed mechanism is that the internally released auristatin E can diffuse out of the killed targeted cell and then kill CD30-negative cells in close proximity to those that have internalized and processed the conjugate.

Taken together, CD30 proved to be the most specific marker for HRS cells of CHL and, furthermore, of the pathognomonic tumor cells of the ALCL. The identification of the CD30 antigen and its sequence analysis contributed significantly to the clarification of the origin of the HRS cells. More than 25 years later, CD30 could be exploited as a therapeutic target by development of an anti-CD30-antibody-drug-conjugate (Senter and colleagues elsewhere in this issue) that has a high potential and specific antilymphoma cell activity without having the limitations of the first-generation conjugates.

REFERENCES

1. Sternberg C. Über eine eigenartige unter dem Bilde der Pseudoleukamie verlaufende Tuberculose des lymphatischen Apparates. Ztschr Heilk 1898;19:21–90.
2. Reed D. On the pathological changes in Hodgkin's disease, with special reference to its relation to tuberculosis. Johns Hopkins Hosp Rep 1902;10:133–96.
3. Stein H, Delsol G, Pileri SA, et al. Classical Hodgkin lymphoma. WHO classification of tumours of haematopoietic and lymphoid tissues. Lyon (France): IARC; 2008.
4. Zech L, Haglund U, Nilsson K, et al. Characteristic chromosomal abnormalities in biopsies and lymphoid-cell lines from patients with Burkitt and non-Burkitt lymphomas. Int J Cancer 1976;17(1):47–56.
5. Kaplan HS, Gartner S. "Sternberg-Reed" giant cells of Hodgkin's disease: cultivation in vitro, heterotransplantation, and characterization as neoplastic macrophages. Int J Cancer 1977;19(4):511–25.

6. Schaadt M, Fonatsch C, Kirchner H, et al. Establishment of a malignant, Epstein-Barr-virus (EBV)-negative cell line from the pleura effusion of a patient with Hodgkin's disease. Blut 1979;38(2):185–90.

7. Schaadt M, Diehl V, Stein H, et al. Two neoplastic cell lines with unique features derived from Hodgkin's disease. Int J Cancer 1980;26(6):723–31 J Cancer Res Clin Oncol 1981;101(1):125–34.

8. Long JC, Zamecnik PC, Aisenberg AC, et al. Tissue culture studies in Hodgkin's disease: morphologic, cytogenetic, cell surface, and enzymatic properties of cultures derived from splenic tumors. J Exp Med 1977;145:1484–500.

9. Harris NL, Gang DL, Quay SC, et al. Contamination of Hodgkin's disease cell cultures. Nature 1981;289(5795):228–30.

10. Stein H, Gerdes J, Kirchner H, et al. Immunohistological analysis of Hodgkin's and Sternberg-Reed cells: detection of a new antigen and evidence for selective IgG uptake in the absence of B cell, T cell and histiocytic markers. J Cancer Res Clin Oncol 1981;101(1):125–34, Int J Cancer 1980;26(6):723–31.

11. Stein H, Gerdes J, Kirchner H, et al. Hodgkin and Sternberg-Reed cell antigen(s) detected by an antiserum to a cell line (L428) derived from Hodgkin's disease. Int J Cancer 1981;28(4):425–9.

12. Gerdes J, Schwab U, Lemke H, et al. Production of a mouse monoclonal antibody reactive with a human nuclear antigen associated with cell proliferation. Int J Cancer 1983;31:13–20.

13. Gerdes J, Lemke H, Baisch H, et al. Cell cycle analysis of a cell proliferation associated human nuclear antigen defined by the monoclonal antibody Ki-67. J Immunol 1984;133:1710–5.

14. Schwab U, Stein H, Gerdes J, et al. Production of a monoclonal antibody specific for Hodgkin and Sternberg-Reed cells of Hodgkin's lymphoma and a subset of normal lymphoid cells. Nature 1982;299:65–7.

15. Stein H, Gerdes J, Schwab U, et al. Identification of Hodgkin and Sternberg-Reed cells as a unique cell type derived from a newly detected small cell population. Int J Cancer 1982;30:445–59.

16. Stein H, Mason DY, Gerdes J, et al. The expression of the Hodgkin's disease-associated antigen Ki-1 in reactive and neoplastic lymphoid tissue. Evidence that Reed-Sternberg cells and histiocytic malignancies are derived from activated lymphoid cells. Blood 1985;66:848–58.

17. Stein H, Foss HD, Dürkop H, et al. CD30(+) anaplastic large cell lymphoma: a review of its histopathologic, genetic, and clinical features. Blood 2000;96(12): 3681–95 [review].

18. Schwarting R, Gerdes J, Dürkop H, et al. Ber-H2: a new anti-Ki-1 (CD30) monoclonal antibody directed at a formol-resistant epitope. Blood 1989;74(5):1678–89.

19. Schwarting R, Gerdes J, Stein H. Ber-H2: a new monoclonal antibody of the Ki-1 family for the detection of Hodgkin's disease in formaldehyde-fixed tissue sections (A2.13). In: McMichael AJ, editor. Leucocyte typing III, white cell differentiation antigens. Oxford (United Kingdom), New York, Tokyo: Oxford University Press; 1987. p. 574–5.

20. Froese P, Lemke H, Gerdes J, et al. Biochemical characterization and biosynthesis of the Ki-1 antigen in Hodgkin-derived and virus-transformed human B and T lymphoid cell lines. J Immunol 1987;139:2081–7.

21. Josimovic-Alasevic O, Dürkop H, Schwarting R, et al. Ki-1 (CD30) antigen is released by Ki-1 positive tumor cells in vitro and in vivo. I. Partial characterization of soluble Ki-1 antigen and detection of the antigen in cell culture supernatants

and in serum by an enzyme-linked immunosorbent assay. Eur J Immunol 1989; 19:157–62.

22. Pizzolo G, Vinante F, Chilosi M, et al. Serum levels of soluble CD30 molecule (Ki-1 antigen) in Hodgkin's Disease. Relationship with disease activity and clinical stage. Br J Haematol 1990;75:282–4.

23. Dürkop H, Latza U, Hummel M, et al. Molecular cloning and expression of a new member of the nerve growth factor receptor family that is characteristic for Hodgkin's disease. Cell 1992;68(3):421–7.

24. Fonatsch C, Latza U, Dürkop H, et al. Assignment of the human CD30 (Ki-1) Gene (hgCD30) to 1p36. Genomics 1992;14:825–6.

25. Küppers R, Rajewsky K, Zhao M, et al. Hodgkin disease: Hodgkin and Reed-Sternberg cells picked from histological sections show clonal immunoglobulin gene rearrangements and appear to be derived from B cells at various stages of development. Proc Natl Acad Sci U S A 1994;91(23):10962–6.

26. Marafioti T, Hummel M, Foss HD, et al. Hodgkin and Reed-Sternberg cells represent an expansion of a single clone originating from a germinal center B-cell with functional immunoglobulin gene rearrangements but defective immunoglobulin transcription. Blood 2000;95(4):1443–50.

27. Falini B, Flenghi L, Fedeli L, et al. In vivo targeting of Hodgkin and Reed-Sternberg cells of Hodgkin's disease with monoclonal antibody Ber-H2 (CD30): immunohistological evidence. Br J Haematol 1992;82:38–45.

28. Ansell SM, Horwitz SM, Engert A, et al. Phase I/II study of an anti-CD30 monoclonal antibody (MDX-060) in Hodgkin's lymphoma and anaplastic large-cell lymphoma. J Clin Oncol 2007;25(19):2764–9.

29. Bartlett NL, Younes A, Carabasi MH, et al. A phase 1 multidose study of SGN-30 immunotherapy in patients with refractory or recurrent CD30+ hematologic malignancies. Blood 2008;111(4):1848–54.

30. Falini B, Bolognesi A, Flenghi L, et al. Response of refractory Hodgkin's disease to monoclonal anti-CD30 immunotoxin. Lancet 1992;339:1195–6.

31. Doronina SO, Toki BE, Torgov MY, et al. Development of potent monoclonal antibody auristatin conjugates for cancer therapy. Nat Biotechnol 2003;21(7):778–84.

32. Sanderson RJ, Hering MA, James SF, et al. In vivo drug-linker stability of an anti-CD30 dipeptide-linked auristatin immunoconjugate. Clin Cancer Res 2005;11(2 Pt 1):843–52.

33. Okeley NM, Miyamoto JB, Zhang X, et al. Intracellular activation of SGN-35, a potent anti-CD30 antibody-drug conjugate. Clin Cancer Res 2010;16(3):888–97.

Advancing Antibody Drug Conjugation

From the Laboratory to a Clinically Approved Anticancer Drug

Nicole M. Okeley, PhD*, Stephen C. Alley, PhD,
Peter D. Senter, PhD

KEYWORDS

- Immunotherapy • Chemotherapeutic • Monoclonal antibody • Tumor
- Drug delivery • Targeting

KEY POINTS

- The concept of using monoclonal antibodies for delivering drugs to cancer cells has been explored for decades, with early work surrounding nonspecific targets and drugs with low potencies.
- These studies underscored the importance of critical parameters, such as antigen and tumor target selection, linker stability, drug potency, pharmacokinetics, and conjugation methodology, in developing effective antibody drug conjugates with acceptable safety profiles.
- Brentuximab vedotin represents the culmination of much research and development activities in which many of these parameters were addressed.
- The drug received accelerated approval for the treatment of relapsed Hodgkin lymphoma and systemic anaplastic large cell lymphoma.

Antibody–drug conjugates (ADCs) for cancer therapy are designed for the specific delivery of cytotoxic agents to tumor tissues, ideally allowing for selective ablation while sparing normal cells from chemotherapeutic damage. The success of an ADC is driven by several factors, not least of which is the choice of appropriate antigen and tumor target, the monoclonal antibody (mAb) used for delivery, the cytotoxic agent attached to the mAb, and the linker and conjugation technology used to join the 2 components (**Fig. 1**).[1–3] The highly specific binding interaction between the mAb and the antigen of interest, and the expression profile of the antigen, are primary drivers of preferential delivery to tumor cells. Drug potency and the mode and multiplicity of attachment

Disclosure of Relationships: The authors are employees and shareholders of Seattle Genetics.
Seattle Genetics Inc, 21823 30th Drive Southeast, Bothell, WA 98021, USA
* Corresponding author.
E-mail address: nokeley@seagen.com

Hematol Oncol Clin N Am 28 (2014) 13–25
http://dx.doi.org/10.1016/j.hoc.2013.10.009
0889-8588/14/$ – see front matter © 2014 Elsevier Inc. All rights reserved.

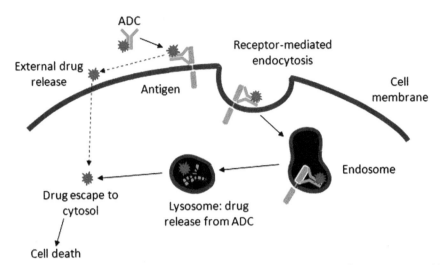

Fig. 1. Mechanism of action of ADCs. The ADC binds to tumor cell surface antigens and is taken up within cells through a process known as *receptor-mediated endocytosis*. On entry into degradative compartments such as lysosomes, the drug can be released by linker hydrolysis or antibody degradation. Cell death occurs once the drug binds to its target. (*From* Alley SC, Jeger S, Lyon, et al. Empowered antibodies for cancer therapy. In: Kratz F, Senter P, Steinhagen H, editors. Drug delivery in oncology: from basic research to cancer therapy. Weinheim (Germany): Wiley-VCH Verlag GmbH & Co. KGaA; 2011. p. 296; with permission.)

to the mAb are also strong determinants in achieving specific cell kill. All of these factors were addressed in the development of brentuximab vedotin (ADCETRIS), an ADC composed of an anti-CD30 mAb (cAC10) linked to monomethyl auristatin E (MMAE) through a protease-cleavable linker. Brentuximab vedotin received accelerated approval by the U.S. Food and Drug Administration for the treatment of relapsed Hodgkin lymphoma and systemic anaplastic large cell lymphoma (ALCL).[4–7] This article details some of the technological advancements and preclinical and clinical findings that led to the generation of this drug.

THE CD30 TARGET ANTIGEN

Cancer cells often overexpress cell surface antigens that distinguish them from normal tissues and allow for the use of targeting reagents for therapeutic intervention.[5] Many of these antigens have been exploited using mAbs designed to recognize them, bind, and elicit selective cell kill because of effector function and signaling activities. To date, 9 mAbs directed against target antigens on leukemias, lymphomas, tumor-infiltrating lymphocytes, and solid tumor malignancies have been clinically approved **(Table 1)**.[8,9] The clinical impact of these approved agents has spawned great interest in exploiting other antigens that are selectively expressed within tumors. CD30 is an example of a highly desirable antigen for targeted therapy, because of minimal normal tissue expression coupled with high expression on some human cancers.[10–12] For example, this antigen is highly expressed on the Reed-Sternberg cells of Hodgkin lymphoma and on systemic ALCL tumor cells. CD30 is also observed on cutaneous T-cell lymphoma and other select lymphoid tumors and some malignancies, including germ cell cancers.[13,14] Its normal physiologic expression is otherwise thought to be limited

Table 1
Unconjugated monoclonal antibodies approved for cancer

Target	Antibody	Therapeutic Indication	First U.S. Approval
CD20	Rituximab	Non-Hodgkin's lymphoma	1997
CD20	Ofatumumab	Chronic lymphocytic leukemia	2009
Her2	Trastuzumab	Breast cancer	1998
Her2	Pertuzumab	Breast cancer	2012
CD52	Alemtuzumab	Chronic lymphocytic leukemia	2001
EGFR	Cetuximab	Colon cancer	2004
EGFR	Panitumumab	Colon cancer	2006
VEGF	Bevacizumab	Colon cancer	2004
CTLA-4	Ipilimumab	Melanoma	2011

to activated T and B cells.[15,16] CD30 is a tumor necrosis factor receptor (TNFR) super-family member, which stimulates apoptosis via TNFR-associated factor 2 degradation.[17,18] Because of its expression profile and its role in the regulation of cell survival, considerable attention has been given to CD30 as a target both for anti-CD30 mAbs and for ADCs. Several studies have been reported for anti-CD30–based therapies, including work with an unconjugated mAb,[19,20] and anti-CD30–toxin conjugates.[21–24] The unconjugated anti-CD30 mAb, cAC10,[14] had promising preclinical activity profiles based on its ability to retard tumor outgrowth through antibody-dependent cellular phagocytosis (ADCP)[25] and signaling activities,[14,26] However, unconjugated cAC10 failed to show convincing clinical efficacy.[19] Much more potent anti-CD30–based reagents were generated with a mAb-ricin A chain conjugate[21,22] and a mAb-saporin conjugate.[23,24] Although these conjugates had very promising in vitro and in vivo activities, they, like many other conjugates such as these, failed to generate convincing clinical efficacy, mostly because of immunogenicity and issues with respect to targeted delivery. Taken together, these studies provided strong preclinical data supporting CD30 as a target for an antibody-based therapy, but indicated that improvements were needed to effectively exploit the presence of this antigen on cancer cells.

DEVELOPMENT OF THE DRUG-LINKER COMPONENT FOR A TARGETED ANTI-CD30 THERAPEUTIC

The concept of using mAbs for delivering drugs to tumor cells was proposed long before tumor-selective mAbs were available. With the advent of newer technologies for the generation of selective, nonimmunogenic mAbs, the field began to be extensively explored using approved anticancer drugs, such as doxorubicin and vinca alkaloids. Clinical trials with drugs such as BR96-doxorubicin[27] highlighted some underlying weaknesses of this approach,[28] which included toxicity from normal tissue antigen expression; low potency of the drug component, requiring high doses to be administered; and the instability of the linker used between the drug and the mAb, resulting in much of the drug being lost within the first few days of administration.[29] To overcome some of these issues, attention turned to the use of highly potent cytotoxins targeted with mAbs that displayed higher degrees of tumor specificity. Gemtuzumab ozogamicin (Mylotarg) was one such agent, which incorporated a high-potency drug component (calicheamicin), conjugated to an antibody (anti-CD33) that displayed significant specificity for antigens expressed on acute myelogenous leukemia. Although the agent was found to be clinically active,[6,30–32] the utility of the drug may have been hampered by the instability of the linker,[33] the susceptibility of the drug to multidrug resistance,[34] and the presence of large amounts of unconjugated antibody in the drug product.[35] Although gemtuzumab ozogamicin was being developed and investigated, continued efforts with highly potent immunotoxins continued, but the efforts were thwarted because of immunogenicity and toxicity.[36–38] Thus, a newer-generation ADC technology required the development of potent drugs that were nonimmunogenic, and could be conjugated to highly selective antitumor antibodies through linker technologies that were more stable than those used previously.

In generating an appropriate drug for ADCs, the authors focused attention on totally synthetic drugs that could be tailor-made for drug delivery. This research led to the development of MMAE (**Fig. 2**), a synthetic analog of dolastatin 10, which was one of several toxic natural products isolated from the Indian Ocean sea hare, *Dolabella auricularia*.[39–41] MMAE exerts its anticancer activity through the inhibition of tubulin polymerization. Some of the features that make MMAE appropriate as the cytotoxic drug component of an ADC include a high potency against a broad array of tumor cell lines; its high water solubility, which helps circumvent ADC aggregation; its stability under physiologic conditions; and, importantly, an intentionally built-in site for stable linker attachment to enable mAb conjugation.[42–44]

A great deal of research has surrounded how MMAE could be effectively conjugated to mAbs against cancer cell–surface antigens, with specific attention placed on the cAC10 mAb that recognizes the CD30 antigen on various lymphomas. Historically,

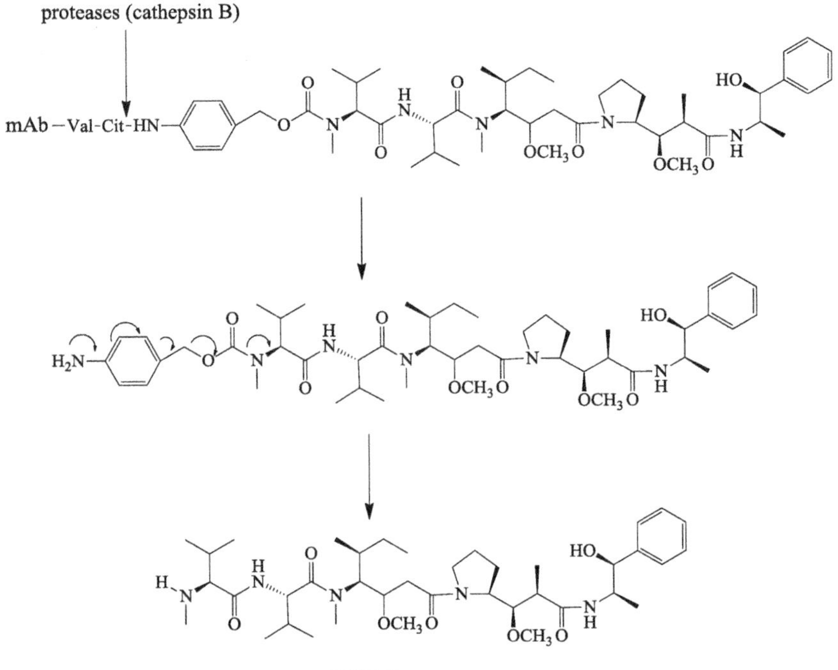

MMAE

Fig. 2. Structure of the auristatin drug-linker component of brentuximab vedotin and the release of the active cytotoxic MMAE on linker hydrolysis by proteases, such as cathepsin B.

there are many ways to attach drugs to mAbs, but most involve the reaction of cysteine side chains with thiol-reactive moieties or lysine side chain amine reactions with active esters.[45] The presence of 4 reducible disulfide bonds within the immuno-globulin G (IgG) structure that covalently link the heavy and light chains together is an attractive feature that allows for selective attachment of drug to up to 8 distinct sites using a thiol-reactive handle. Up to 100 lysines are present in typical IgG1 mAbs, and conjugation to these sites through amine-reactive linkers results in a great deal more heterogeneity than that obtained using cysteines generated through disulfide reduc-tion (**Fig. 3**).[46]

The number of drugs conjugated to reduced antibody disulfides can be optimized using partial reduction techniques. Although in vitro cytotoxicity potency increases with increased multiplicity of drug conjugation, in vivo potency is actually dimin-ished.[43] This paradoxic observation can be explained by ADC pharmacokinetics, in which it was found that longer circulation half-lives were obtained with drug loadings of 2 or 4 per mAb compared with fully loaded ADCs containing 8 drugs per mAb (**Fig. 4**). Controlling drug substitution to levels that preserve the pharmacokinetic pa-rameters of the parent mAb has generally been found to provide longer tumor expo-sure, better activity, and reduced toxicity.

Selective delivery of a highly potent drug to tumors is also dependent on the use of a linker technology that can provide conditional stability, preventing release of the drug in circulation but allowing its discharge after tumor binding and ADC internalization

Homogeneous products   **Heterogeneous products**

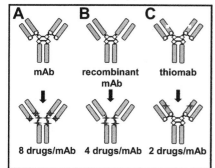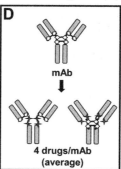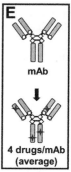

◇ cys   − disulfide   ＋ drug

Fig. 3. Various drug conjugation strategies. ADCs can have high homogeneity. (*A*) mAbs are fully reduced and 8 drugs are added to the 8 reduced interchain cysteines (cys).[27,42,56] (*B*) A recombinant mAb with 4 interchain cysteines mutated to alanine yields an ADC with 4 drugs per mAb after full reduction and conjugation.[55] (*C*) Additional unpaired cysteines can be genetically introduced into the mAb, requiring full reduction and reoxidation of the inter-chain disulfides, followed by drug conjugation to yield 2 drugs per mAb.[61] Heterogeneous products are obtained when (*D*) ADC mixtures containing an average of 4 drugs per mAb are formed by partial reduction of mAb disulfides followed by conjugation.[44,46] ADCs with the greatest structural complexity (*E*) are formed by alkylating lysines with a drug-linker or alkylating lysines with a maleimide-containing linker followed by conjugation to a thiol-containing drug yielding an average 2 to 4 drugs per mAb. These ADCs will have drugs dispersed among many mAb lysines.[55,62–64] (*From* Alley SC, Jeger S, Lyon, et al. Empowered antibodies for cancer therapy. In: Kratz F, Senter P, Steinhagen H, editors. Drug delivery in oncology: from basic research to cancer therapy. Weinheim (Germany): Wiley-VCH Verlag GmbH & Co. KGaA; 2011. p. 298; with permission.)

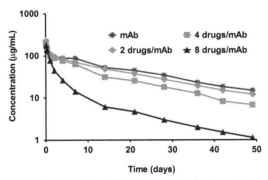

Fig. 4. Pharmacokinetics of ADCs with different drug loads. Unconjugated cAC10 and puri-fied cAC10-Val-Cit-MMAE with 2, 4, or 8 drugs per mAb were injected into mice and the mAb concentration was measured using enzyme-linked immunosorbent assay. (*From* Ham-blett KJ, Senter PD, Chace DF, et al. Effects of drug loading on the antitumor activity of a monoclonal antibody drug conjugate. Clin Cancer Res 2004;10:7068; with permission.)

(see **Fig. 1**). Several different linker technologies exist, with varying stability profiles, including hydrazones, disulfide linkers, protease-cleavable dipeptide linkers, and thi-oether linkers.[2] Drug release from hydrazones and disulfide linkers can be achieved under intracellular conditions, such as the low-pH environment in lysosomes or the reducing environment of the cytosol.[47] For example, the ADC gemtuzumab ozogami-cin contains an acid-labile hydrazone linking the calicheamicin-derived cytotoxic component to the CD33 mAb.[48] However, both acid-labile hydrazone linkers and disulfide-based linkers are unstable in plasma, with half-lives in plasma ranging be-tween 1 and 3 days.[33,42] An alternative method for intracellular drug release is through the use of linkers predominantly cleaved by specific lysosomal proteases, such as the valine-citrulline dipeptide linkers.[49] This type of linkage imparts greater stability in plasma and increased exposure to the conjugated drug after intravenous delivery than the hydrazone or disulfide linkages.[50] Brentuximab vedotin is an ADC that uses a cleavable valine-citrulline dipeptide linker to facilitate release of MMAE.[6] The ADC is composed of an average of 4 molecules of MMAE attached to cAC10 interchain cysteine residues through the protease-cleavable maleimidocaproyl-valine-citrulline-para-aminobenzyl linker (Val-Cit). Typical preparations of brentuximab vedotin contain less than 2% aggregated protein and bind to CD30 with unaltered affinity (3 nM) compared with the unconjugated antibody.[5,43,51]

EVALUATION OF BRENTUXIMAB VEDOTIN ACTIVITY IN VITRO

Brentuximab vedotin was evaluated for potency on cell lines in vitro, comparing activ-ity on CD30+ Hodgkin lymphoma and ALCL tumor cells and CD30− tumor lines. Potent activity was observed on antigen positive cell lines, whereas no activity was detectable in antigen-negative cells. Half-maximal inhibitory concentration (IC_{50}) values on CD30+ cell lines were in the range of 3 to 50 pM (0.5–8.0 ng/mL) (**Fig. 5**A).[5,43,51] Non–CD30-expressing cells were approximately 1000 times less sen-sitive to the effects of the ADC, demonstrating its immunologic specificity.

The ADC delivers its payload through binding to the cell surface, followed by receptor-mediated endocytosis (see **Fig. 1**). The endocytic vesicle matures into a lyso-some, where proteolytic activity can both cleave the designed proteolytically labile bond in the linker and degrade the antibody itself. When the peptide bond of the

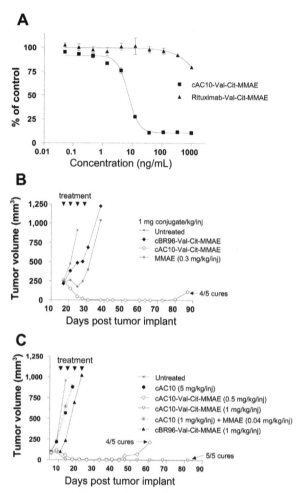

Fig. 5. In vitro and in vivo activity of auristatin ADCs. (*A*) In vitro ADC cytotoxicity was evaluated by treating CD30+ KARPAS 299 cells with CD30-binding cAC10-Val-Cit-MMAE and control nonbinding rituximab-Val-Cit-MMAE for 96 hours. (*B*) In vivo ADC activity was evaluated by treating CD30+ KARPAS 299 xenografts in SCID mice with CD30-binding cAC10-Val-Cit-MMAE and nonbinding cBR96-Val-Cit-MMAE. (*C*) In vivo ADC activity was evaluated by treating CD30+ KARPAS 299 xenografts in SCID mice with CD30-binding cAC10-Val-Cit-MMAE and a molar equivalent mixture of cAC10 and unconjugated MMAE. (*Data from* Refs.[42,56]; and *From* Alley SC, Jeger S, Lyon, et al. Empowered antibodies for cancer therapy. In: Kratz F, Senter P, Steinhagen H, editors. Drug delivery in oncology: from basic research to cancer therapy. Weinheim (Germany): Wiley-VCH Verlag GmbH & Co. KGaA; 2011. p. 305; with permission.)

linker is cleaved, MMAE is released through a self-immolative reaction of the spacer para-aminobenzyl group. The drug can then diffuse within the cell, where it eventually binds to microtubules, or can diffuse out of the cell. Studies confirmed that cysteine proteases within the cell are involved with MMAE release, because cellular treatment with protease inhibitors reduced the in vitro activity of cAC10-Val-Cit-MMAE.[52] Antigen-mediated generation of MMAE in antigen-positive cells treated with brentuximab vedotin was previously demonstrated, resulting in high cellular accumulation of MMAE together with some diffusion of the internally released MMAE out of the cell into the culture medium.[53] It was also shown that antigen-negative cells cultured with the ADC did not generate MMAE, demonstrating the immunologic specificity of ADC drug delivery. The diffusion of internally released MMAE out of antigen-positive cells points to potential activity on cells that are close to those that have internalized and processed the targeted ADC. This bystander activity was confirmed in co-culture assays between CD30+ and CD30– cells treated with brentuximab vedotin.[53] Bystander activity has also been observed with a maytasine drug conjugate using an alternative linker technology.[54] The importance that this activity plays in the activity of brentuximab vedotin is the subject on ongoing research.

EVALUATION OF BRENTUXIMAB VEDOTIN ACTIVITY IN VIVO

The activity of brentuximab vedotin was evaluated in immunologically deficient mice with human Hodgkin lymphoma[55] and anaplastic large-cell lymphoma xenografts (see **Fig. 5**B, C).[42,43,56] The studies demonstrated that the anti-CD30 ADC was active at 1 to 3 mg/kg, which was well below the maximum tolerated dose of approximately 100 mg/kg. The effects were immunologically specific, because non–antigen-expressing cells were much less impacted by treatment.[43] A favorable half-life of the ADC was observed, which was 14.0 days in mice compared with 16.7 days for the unconjugated antibody.[43] Ex vivo studies with Val-Cit-MMAE–conjugated ADC revealed that very little released MMAE was generated in human or mouse plasma with only 2% or 5%, respectively, of the conjugated drug being detected after 10 days at 37°C.[50] The stability of the drug-linker in circulation was also investigated and found to be promising in mice and cynomolgous monkeys, with drug-linker half-lives of 6.0 to 9.6 days, respectively.[50] The loss of drug-linker from the antibody was determined to result from reversibility of the maleimide linkage.[57] Thus, brentuximab vedotin seems to have improved stability characteristics compared with the earlier-generation hydrazone-based ADCs.

CLINICAL EXPERIENCE WITH BRENTUXIMAB VEDOTIN

Brentuximab vedotin entered clinical trials in 2006, starting with a single-agent dose-escalation trial in patients with CD30-positive malignancies.[58] When given every 3 weeks, a maximum tolerated dose of 1.8 mg/kg was established. For all 45 patients in the trial, a 38% objective response rate was seen, and a 24% complete response rate. Weekly dosing was explored in a second single-agent trial, and a slightly lower maximum tolerated dose of 1.2 mg/kg was obtained.[59] For all 44 patients in this trial, a 59% objective response rate was seen, with a 34% complete response rate. The most common adverse events in both trials were fatigue, pyrexia, diarrhea, nausea, neutropenia, sensory peripheral neuropathy, and arthralgia.

Based on these results, 2 single-arm, pivotal phase 2 trials were conducted in patients with relapsed or refractory Hodgkin lymphoma[7] and ALCL[4] using the 1.8 mg/kg dose every 3 weeks. Objective responses were observed in 75% and 86% of patients, with complete remissions observed in 34% and 57% of patients with Hodgkin lymphoma and ALCL, respectively. The most common adverse events in these studies were peripheral sensory neuropathy, nausea, fatigue, neutropenia, and diarrhea. In separate clinical trials, brentuximab vedotin was also evaluated clinically for drug–drug interactions and route of excretion. Patients were treated with brentuximab vedotin and a CYP3A substrate (midazolam), inducer (rifampin), or inhibitor (ketoconazole), and pharmacokinetics were evaluated.[60] Although midazolam

Table 2
Ongoing phase 3 trials of brentuximab vedotin

Trial	Therapeutic Area	Combination
ECHELON-1	Newly diagnosed advanced classical Hodgkin lymphoma	AVD (doxorubicin, vinblastine, and dacarbazine)
ECHELON-2	Newly diagnosed mature T-cell lymphomas	CHP (cyclophosphamide, doxorubicin, prednisone)
AETHERA	High risk of residual Hodgkin lymphoma after autologous stem cell transplant	None
ALCANZA	Relapsed CD30+ cutaneous T-cell lymphoma (primary cutaneous ALCL, mycosis fungoides)	None

exposures were not affected by brentuximab vedotin and brentuximab vedotin exposures were not affected by rifampin or ketoconazole, MMAE exposures were lower with rifampin and higher with ketoconazole, suggesting that brentuximab vedotin and MMAE are neither inhibitors nor inducers of CYP3A, but that MMAE is a substrate of CYP3A. The primary route of excretion was found to be via feces, with MMAE recovered mostly unchanged.[60]

In August 2011, brentuximab vedotin received accelerated approval for the treatment of relapsed Hodgkin lymphoma and systemic ALCL. The drug is currently being evaluated in phase 3 trials in Hodgkin lymphoma and T-cell lymphomas, some of which include combination with standard chemotherapy (**Table 2**). Many earlier stage clinical trials are underway that apply the drug-linker technology developed in brentuximab vedotin to other disease indications (**Table 3**). In the next few years, data from these trials will provide significant insights into how the technology can be extended.

Table 3
Auristatin antibody drug conjugates in clinical development

Drug	Status	Therapeutic Area	Target
CDX-011	Phase 2	Breast cancer	GPNMB
PSMA ADC	Phase 2	Prostate	PSMA
DCDT2980S	Phase 2	Non-Hodgkin's lymphoma	CD22
DCDS4501A	Phase 2	Non-Hodgkin's lymphoma	CD79b
SGN-75	Phase 1b	Renal cell carcinoma	CD70
AGS-16M8F	Phase 1	Renal cell carcinoma	AGS-16
ASG-22ME	Phase 1	Solid tumors	Nectin-4
ABT-414	Phase 1/2	Squamous cell tumors	EGFR
RG7450	Phase 1	Prostate cancer	STEAP1
DMUC5754A	Phase 1	Ovarian cancer	MUC16
RG7599	Phase 1	Ovarian, lung cancer	NaPi2b
MLN0264	Phase 1	Colorectal cancer	GCC
RG7636	Phase 1	Melanoma	ETBR
SGN-CD19A	Phase 1	Acute lymphocytic leukemia, non-Hodgkin's lymphoma	CD19

REFERENCES

1. Alley SC, Okeley NM, Senter PD. Antibody-drug conjugates: targeted drug delivery for cancer. Curr Opin Chem Biol 2010;14:529–37.
2. Chari RV. Targeted cancer therapy: conferring specificity to cytotoxic drugs. Acc Chem Res 2008;41:98–107.
3. Senter PD. Potent antibody drug conjugates for cancer therapy. Curr Opin Chem Biol 2009;13:235–44.
4. Pro B, Advani R, Brice P, et al. Brentuximab vedotin (SGN-35) in patients with relapsed or refractory systemic anaplastic large-cell lymphoma: results of a phase II study. J Clin Oncol 2012;30:2190–6.
5. Senter PD, Sievers EL. The discovery and development of brentuximab vedotin for use in relapsed Hodgkin lymphoma and systemic anaplastic large cell lymphoma. Nat Biotechnol 2012;30:631–7.
6. Sievers EL, Senter PD. Antibody-drug conjugates in cancer therapy. Annu Rev Med 2013;64:15–29.
7. Younes A, Gopal AK, Smith SE, et al. Results of a pivotal phase II study of brentuximab vedotin for patients with relapsed or refractory Hodgkin's lymphoma. J Clin Oncol 2012;30:2183–9.
8. Mullard A. Maturing antibody-drug conjugate pipeline hits 30. Nat Rev Drug Discov 2013;12:329–32.
9. Nelson AL, Dhimolea E, Reichert JM. Development trends for human monoclonal antibody therapeutics. Nat Rev Drug Discov 2010;9:767–74.
10. Chiarle R, Podda A, Prolla G, et al. CD30 in normal and neoplastic cells. Clin Immunol 1999;90:157–64.
11. Schwab U, Stein H, Gerdes J, et al. Production of a monoclonal antibody specific for Hodgkin and Sternberg-Reed cells of Hodgkin's disease and a subset of normal lymphoid cells. Nature 1982;299:65–7.
12. Stein H, Mason DY, Gerdes J, et al. The expression of the Hodgkin's disease associated antigen Ki-1 in reactive and neoplastic lymphoid tissue: evidence that Reed-Sternberg cells and histiocytic malignancies are derived from activated lymphoid cells. Blood 1985;66:848–58.
13. Deutsch YE, Tadmor T, Podack ER, et al. CD30: an important new target in hematologic malignancies. Leuk Lymphoma 2011;52:1641–54.
14. Wahl AF, Klussman K, Thompson JD, et al. The anti-CD30 monoclonal antibody SGN-30 promotes growth arrest and DNA fragmentation in vitro and affects antitumor activity in models of Hodgkin's disease. Cancer Res 2002;62:3736–42.
15. Falini B, Pileri S, Pizzolo G, et al. CD30 (Ki-1) molecule: a new cytokine receptor of the tumor necrosis factor receptor superfamily as a tool for diagnosis and immunotherapy. Blood 1995;85:1–14.
16. Stein H, Foss HD, Durkop H, et al. CD30(+) anaplastic large cell lymphoma: a review of its histopathologic, genetic, and clinical features. Blood 2000;96:3681–95.
17. Duckett CS, Thompson CB. CD30-dependent degradation of TRAF2: implications for negative regulation of TRAF signaling and the control of cell survival. Genes Dev 1997;11:2810–21.
18. Durkop H, Latza U, Hummel M, et al. Molecular cloning and expression of a new member of the nerve growth factor receptor family that is characteristic for Hodgkin's disease. Cell 1992;68:421–7.
19. Ansell SM, Horwitz SM, Engert A, et al. Phase I/II study of an anti-CD30 monoclonal antibody (MDX-060) in Hodgkin's lymphoma and anaplastic large-cell lymphoma. J Clin Oncol 2007;25:2764–9.

20. Forero-Torres A, Leonard JP, Younes A, et al. A phase II study of SGN-30 (anti-CD30 mAb) in Hodgkin lymphoma or systemic anaplastic large cell lymphoma. Br J Haematol 2009;146:171–9.
21. Schnell R, Borchmann P, Staak JO, et al. Clinical evaluation of ricin A-chain immunotoxins in patients with Hodgkin's lymphoma. Ann Oncol 2003;14:729–36.
22. Schnell R, Staak O, Borchmann P, et al. A phase I study with an anti-CD30 ricin A-chain immunotoxin (Ki-4.dgA) in patients with refractory CD30+ Hodgkin's and non-Hodgkin's lymphoma. Clin Cancer Res 2002;8:1779–86.
23. Tazzari PL, Bolognesi A, de Totero D, et al. Ber-H2 (anti-CD30)-saporin immunotoxin: a new tool for the treatment of Hodgkin's disease and CD30+ lymphoma: in vitro evaluation. Br J Haematol 1992;81:203–11.
24. Falini B, Bolognesi A, Flenghi L, et al. Response of refractory Hodgkin's disease to monoclonal anti-CD30 immunotoxin. Lancet 1992;339:1195–6.
25. Oflazoglu E, Stone IJ, Gordon KA, et al. Macrophages contribute to the antitumor activity of the anti-CD30 antibody SGN-30. Blood 2007;110:4370–2.
26. Cerveny CG, Law CL, McCormick RS, et al. Signaling via the anti-CD30 mAb SGN-30 sensitizes Hodgkin's disease cells to conventional chemotherapeutics. Leukemia 2005;19:1648–55.
27. Trail PA, Willner D, Lasch SJ, et al. Cure of xenografted human carcinomas by BR96-doxorubicin immunoconjugates. Science 1993;261:212–5.
28. Saleh MN, Sugarman S, Murray J, et al. Phase I trial of the anti-Lewis Y drug immunoconjugate BR96-doxorubicin in patients with Lewis Y-expressing epithelial tumors. J Clin Oncol 2000;18:2282–92.
29. Mosure KW, Henderson AJ, Klunk LJ, et al. Disposition of conjugate-bound and free doxorubicin in tumor-bearing mice following administration of a BR96-doxorubicin immunoconjugate (BMS 182248). Cancer Chemother Pharmacol 1997;40:251–8.
30. Burnett AK, Hills RK, Hunter AE, et al. The addition of gemtuzumab ozogamicin to low-dose Ara-C improves remission rate but does not significantly prolong survival in older patients with acute myeloid leukaemia: results from the LRF AML14 and NCRI AML16 pick-a-winner comparison. Leukemia 2012;27:75–81.
31. Burnett AK, Hills RK, Milligan D, et al. Identification of patients with acute myeloblastic leukemia who benefit from the addition of gemtuzumab ozogamicin: results of the MRC AML15 trial. J Clin Oncol 2011;29:369–77.
32. Castaigne S, Pautas C, Terre C, et al. Effect of gemtuzumab ozogamicin on survival of adult patients with de-novo acute myeloid leukaemia (ALFA-0701): a randomised, open-label, phase 3 study. Lancet 2012;379:1508–16.
33. Boghaert ER, Khandke KM, Sridharan L, et al. Determination of pharmacokinetic values of calicheamicin-antibody conjugates in mice by plasmon resonance analysis of small (5 microl) blood samples. Cancer Chemother Pharmacol 2008;61:1027–35.
34. Walter RB, Gooley TA, van der Velden VH, et al. CD33 expression and P-glycoprotein-mediated drug efflux inversely correlate and predict clinical outcome in patients with acute myeloid leukemia treated with gemtuzumab ozogamicin monotherapy. Blood 2007;109:4168–70.
35. Bross PF, Beitz J, Chen G, et al. Approval summary: gemtuzumab ozogamicin in relapsed acute myeloid leukemia. Clin Cancer Res 2001;7:1490–6.
36. Schnell R, Vitetta E, Schindler J, et al. Clinical trials with an anti-CD25 ricin A-chain experimental and immunotoxin (RFT5-SMPT-dgA) in Hodgkin's lymphoma. Leuk Lymphoma 1998;30:525–37.

37. Thorpe PE, Brown AN, Ross WC, et al. Cytotoxicity acquired by conjugation of an anti-Thy1.1 monoclonal antibody and the ribosome-inactivating protein, gelonin. Eur J Biochem 1981;116:447–54.
38. Vitetta ES, Thorpe PE, Uhr JW. Immunotoxins: magic bullets or misguided missiles? Immunol Today 1993;14:252–9.
39. Pettit G. The isolation and structure of a remarkable marine animal antineoplastic constituent: Dolastatin 10. J Am Chem Soc 1987;109:6883–5.
40. Pettit G. The absolute configuration and synthesis of natural (-)-dolastatin 10. J Am Chem Soc 1989;111:5463–5.
41. Pettit GR, Srirangam JK, Barkoczy J, et al. Antineoplastic agents 365. Dolastatin 10 SAR probes. Anticancer Drug Des 1998;13:243–77.
42. Doronina SO, Toki BE, Torgov MY, et al. Development of potent monoclonal antibody auristatin conjugates for cancer therapy. Nat Biotechnol 2003;21:778–84.
43. Hamblett KJ, Senter PD, Chace DF, et al. Effects of drug loading on the antitumor activity of a monoclonal antibody drug conjugate. Clin Cancer Res 2004;10:7063–70.
44. Sun MM, Beam KS, Cerveny CG, et al. Reduction-alkylation strategies for the modification of specific monoclonal antibody disulfides. Bioconjug Chem 2005;16:1282–90.
45. Hermanson GT. Bioconjugate techniques. San Diego: Academic Press; 1996.
46. Lyon RP, Meyer DL, Setter JR, et al. Conjugation of anticancer drugs through endogenous monoclonal antibody cysteine residues. Methods Enzymol 2012;502:123–38.
47. Erickson HK, Widdison WC, Mayo MF, et al. Tumor delivery and in vivo processing of disulfide-linked and thioether-linked antibody-maytansinoid conjugates. Bioconjug Chem 2010;21:84–92.
48. Hamann PR, Hinman LM, Beyer CF, et al. An anti-CD33 antibody-calicheamicin conjugate for treatment of acute myeloid leukemia. Choice of linker. Bioconjug Chem 2002;13:40–6.
49. Dubowchik GM, Firestone RA. Cathepsin B-sensitive dipeptide prodrugs. 1. A model study of structural requirements for efficient release of doxorubicin. Bioorg Med Chem Lett 1998;8:3341–6.
50. Sanderson RJ, Hering MA, James SF, et al. In vivo drug-linker stability of an anti-CD30 dipeptide-linked auristatin immunoconjugate. Clin Cancer Res 2005;11:843–52.
51. Kim KM, McDonagh CF, Westendorf L, et al. Anti-CD30 diabody-drug conjugates with potent antitumor activity. Mol Cancer Ther 2008;7:2486–97.
52. Sutherland MS, Sanderson RJ, Gordon KA, et al. Lysosomal trafficking and cysteine protease metabolism confer target-specific cytotoxicity by peptide-linked anti-CD30-auristatin conjugates. J Biol Chem 2006;281:10540–7.
53. Okeley NM. Intracellular activation of SGN-35, a potent Anti-CD30 antibody-drug conjugate. Clin Cancer Res 2010;16:888–97.
54. Erickson HK, Park PU, Widdison WC, et al. Antibody-maytansinoid conjugates are activated in targeted cancer cells by lysosomal degradation and linker-dependent intracellular processing. Cancer Res 2006;66:4426–33.
55. McDonagh CF, Turcott E, Westendorf L, et al. Engineered antibody-drug conjugates with defined sites and stoichiometries of drug attachment. Protein Eng Des Sel 2006;19:299–307.
56. Francisco JA, Cerveny CG, Meyer DL, et al. cAC10-vcMMAE, an anti-CD30-monomethyl auristatin E conjugate with potent and selective antitumor activity. Blood 2003;102:1458–65.

57. Alley SC, Benjamin DR, Jeffrey SC, et al. Contribution of linker stability to the activities of anticancer immunoconjugates. Bioconjug Chem 2008;19:759–65.
58. Younes A, Forero-Torres A, Bartlett NL, et al. Objective responses in a phase I dose-escalation study of SGN-35, a novel antibody-drug conjugate (ADC) targeting CD30, in patients with relapsed or refractory Hodgkin lymphoma. J Clin Oncol 2008;26(Suppl). Abstract: 8526.
59. Fanale M, Bartlett NL, Forero-Torres A, et al. The antibody-drug conjugate brentuximab vedotin (SGN-35) induced multiple objective responses in patients with relapsed or refractory CD30-positive lymphomas in a phase 1 weekly dosing study. Presented at the 51st ASH Annual Meeting and Exposition. New Orleans, December 5–8, 2009.
60. Han TH, Gopal AK, Ramchandren R, et al. CYP3A-Mediated drug-drug interaction potential and excretion of Brentuximab Vedotin, an antibody-drug conjugate, in patients with CD30-positive hematologic malignancies. J Clin Pharmacol 2013;53:866–77.
61. Junutula JR, Raab H, Clark S, et al. Site-specific conjugation of a cytotoxic drug to an antibody improves the therapeutic index. Nat Biotechnol 2008;26:925–32.
62. Chari RV, Martell BA, Gross JL, et al. Immunoconjugates containing novel maytansinoids: promising anticancer drugs. Cancer Res 1992;52:127–31.
63. Lu SX, Takach EJ, Solomon M, et al. Mass spectral analyses of labile DOTA-NHS and heterogeneity determination of DOTA or DM1 conjugated anti-PSMA antibody for prostate cancer therapy. J Pharm Sci 2005;94:788–97.
64. Wang L, Amphlett G, Blättler WA, et al. Structural characterization of the maytansinoid-monoclonal antibody immunoconjugate, huN901-DM1, by mass spectrometry. Protein Sci 2005;14:2436–46.

Brentuximab Vedotin for the Treatment of Patients with Hodgkin Lymphoma

Anas Younes, MD

KEYWORDS

- CD30 • Reed-Sternberg • Monoclonal antibody • Antibody-drug conjugate

KEY POINTS

- Brentuximab vedotin, an antibody-drug conjugate that targets CD30, is one of the most active single agents for the treatment of patients with relapsed classic Hodgkin lymphoma.
- Brentuximab vedotin should not be combined with bleomycin, as the combination can cause excessive pulmonary toxicity. When combined with front-line ABVD, bleomycin is eliminated from the regimen.
- The most common brentuximab vedotin toxicity is cumulative but reversible neuropathy.
- Brentuximab vedotin can be safely administered before and after allogeneic stem cell transplant.

INTRODUCTION

CD30 is considered an ideal target for monoclonal antibody therapy for Hodgkin lymphoma (HL), because its expression is highly restricted to the malignant Hodgkin and Reed-Sternberg (HRS) cells.[1] CD30 is a transmembrane receptor that belongs to the tumor necrosis factor receptor superfamily.[2,3] In addition to its membrane-bound form, CD30 can also be shed in a soluble form.[4–6] Over the past 2 decades, several investigators have evaluated the safety and efficacy of a wide range of monoclonal antibodies targeting CD30 in patients with relapsed HL. Results from clinical trials using a variety of naked monoclonal antibodies targeting CD30 have demonstrated an excellent safety profile, but with limited antitumor activity (**Table 1**).[7,8] These disappointing clinical results could be attributed to poor antigen-binding properties of these antibodies, ineffective activation of effector cells, and/or neutralization by high levels of soluble serum CD30.[7–9]

Lymphoma Service, Memorial Sloan-Kettering Cancer Center, New York, NY 10065, USA
E-mail address: younesa@mskcc.org

Hematol Oncol Clin N Am 28 (2014) 27–32
http://dx.doi.org/10.1016/j.hoc.2013.10.005
0889-8588/14/$ – see front matter © 2014 Elsevier Inc. All rights reserved.

hemonc.theclinics.com

Table 1
Results of recent clinical trials targeting CD30 in patients with relapsed classic Hodgkin lymphoma

Drug	Phase of Study	No. of Evaluable Patients	PR	CR	PR + CR
MDX-060	II	63	2	2	4 (6%)
SGN-30	II	38	0	0	0
Xmab2513	I	13	1	0	1 (7%)
SGN-35 (every 3 wk)	I	42	7	10	17 (40%)
SGN-35 (weekly)	I	35	10	6	16 (46%)
Brentuximab vedotin[21]	II	102	41	35	76 (75%)

Abbreviations: CR, complete remission; PR, partial remission.
From Younes A. CD30-targeted antibody therapy. Curr Opin Oncol 2011;23(6):587–93; with permission.

CD30 is internalized, making it a suitable target for antibody-drug conjugate (ADC) treatment strategies. Earlier, custom-made ADCs demonstrated clinical efficacy but also resulted in significant toxicity. More recently, the naked antibody SGN30 was linked to the antitubulin monomethyl auristatin E (MMAE), to generate the ADC brentuximab vedotin (formerly known as SGN35).[10–12]

PHASE I STUDIES

The initial multicenter first-in-man phase I study enrolled 45 patients with relapsed or refractory CD30-positive hematologic cancers, of whom 93% had HL.[13] Although there was no limit to the number of prior regimens, patients were treated with a median of 3 prior regimens, and 73% of the patients had undergone prior autologous stem cell transplantation (ASCT). Patients were treated with escalating doses of brentuximab vedotin (from 0.1 mg/kg to 3.6 mg/kg) in a standard 3 + 3 phase I design. Brentuximab vedotin was administered intravenously, over 30 minutes, every 3 weeks in an outpatient setting. Dose-limiting toxicities included grade-4 thrombocytopenia, grade-3 hyperglycemia, and febrile neutropenia. Based on this phase I study, the recommended dose for the follow-up phase II study was established as 1.8 mg/kg every 3 weeks. Objective responses were observed in 17 patients, including 11 complete remissions (see **Table 1**). When the analysis was restricted to the patients receiving the dose levels of 1.8 mg/kg or greater, 6 of 12 (50%) patients responded, including 4 complete remissions. Using a waterfall plot analysis, tumor regression was observed in 86% of the evaluable patients. The median duration of response was at least 9.7 months.

A second phase I study investigated the safety and tolerability of brentuximab vedotin administered on a weekly schedule for 3 weeks, followed by 1 week of rest.[14] A total of 37 patients (31 had HL) were enrolled and treated. Patients received a median of 3 prior chemotherapy regimens (range 1–8), and 62% previously received an ASCT. The dose-limiting toxicities were grade-3 gastrointestinal (diarrhea and/or vomiting) and grade-4 hyperglycemia. Sixteen (46%) had a major response, with 29% achieving complete remission.

PIVOTAL PHASE II STUDY

Based on the encouraging results that were observed in the phase I studies, a pivotal phase II clinical trial in patients with relapsed HL after receiving ASCT was conducted.[15] Patients received brentuximab vedotin 1.8 mg/kg (capped dose at 180 mg) every 3 weeks by a short 30-minute outpatient intravenous infusion for up to 16 cycles. For those who had a response and an acceptable toxicity profile, up to 16 doses or 1 year of therapy was allowed. Of the 102 patients enrolled, 53% were female and the median age was 31 years (range 15–77 years). Patients had received a median of 3.5 (range 1–13) prior chemotherapy regimens, and all were required to have failed an ASCT. Seventy-one percent had relapsed within 1 year of ASCT. Seventy-six of 102 patients (75%) achieved a major response, of whom 34% achieved complete remission. Overall, 94% had some reduction in their tumor measurements. Responses were rapid, with a median time to treatment response of 5.7 weeks and time to achieving complete remission of 12 weeks. The median duration of response in patients who achieved complete remission was approximately 2 years. The most common treatment-related side effects were peripheral neuropathy (42%), nausea (35%), and fatigue (34%). Neuropathy of grade 3 or higher was seen in 8% of patients and was the most common reason for discontinuation of brentuximab vedotin. The results of brentuximab vedotin single-agent activity compared favorably with the overall response rate using the multiagent chemotherapy regimen of gemcitabine, vinorelbine, and liposomal doxorubicin, but with much lower toxicity.[16] Recent cohort comparison suggested that brentuximab vedotin therapy may have a favorable impact on patient survival, but this will need to be confirmed in a randomized study.[17]

BRENTUXIMAB VEDOTIN IN RELAPSED PRETRANSPLANT AND TRANSPLANT-INELIGIBLE PATIENTS WITH HODGKIN LYMPHOMA

The Food and Drug Administration (FDA)-approved indication for brentuximab vedotin is for the treatment of patients with HL after failure of ASCT or after failure of at least 2 prior multiagent chemotherapy regimens in patients who are not ASCT candidates. Emerging data suggest that introducing brentuximab vedotin in second-line regimens may also be beneficial. Results from an ongoing study using a weekly schedule of brentuximab vedotin at 1.2 mg/kg for 3 weeks in 4 weekly cycles demonstrated that 33% of patients can achieve a positron-emission tomography–negative disease status after 2 cycles of brentuximab vedotin, and therefore were able to proceed to stem cell transplantation without the need for salvage chemotherapy. Randomized studies will be needed to confirm the efficacy of brentuximab vedotin as a single agent or in combination with less toxic chemotherapy regimens before ASCT.

EXPERIENCE WITH BRENTUXIMAB VEDOTIN IN PATIENTS UNDERGOING ALLOGENEIC STEM CELL TRANSPLANTATION

Before the FDA approval of brentuximab vedotin, allogeneic stem cell transplantation was routinely offered to young, healthy patients after failing ASCT. At present, brentuximab vedotin is frequently used as a bridge to an allogeneic stem cell transplant. While this approach may provide high response rates with little toxicity, it remains unclear whether all patients who achieve complete remission after brentuximab vedotin will require consolidation with allogeneic stem cell transplantation.[18] Furthermore, emerging data suggest that up to 30% of patients who achieve complete remission with brentuximab vedotin may have a prolonged duration of remission with a good quality of life. Finally, there are emerging data indicating that retreatment with brentuximab vedotin can be effective, perhaps allowing for a delayed decision regarding immediate need for consolidation with allogeneic stem cell transplantation for selected patients.

There is limited experience with brentuximab vedotin therapy after autologous transplantation as a consolidation strategy, or after relapse from allogeneic stem cell transplantation. A randomized study of brentuximab vedotin versus placebo as adjuvant therapy in patients who received autologous stem cell transplant but at risk for relapsed disease (ATHERA study) has completed accrual of 329 patients. The results of the ATHERA trial will aim to provide valuable information on the role of brentuximab vedotin in this setting. Finally, the safety and efficacy of brentuximab vedotin were recently examined in 25 patients with HL relapsing after allogeneic stem cell transplantation. Treatment was palliative, with an overall response rate of 50% and a median progression-free survival of 7.8 months.

BRENTUXIMAB VEDOTIN IN FRONT-LINE REGIMENS

To improve the cure rate achieved with front-line chemotherapy regimens, brentuximab vedotin was recently combined with the standard ABVD (Adriamycin/Bleomycin/Vinblastine/Dacarbazine) regimen in a phase I study.[19] Initially, escalating doses of brentuximab vedotin (0.6, 0.9, 1.2 mg/kg) were combined with ABVD, given every 2 weeks. Although the clinical efficacy of brentuximab vedotin plus ABVD in the first 25 patients was excellent, up to 40% of the patients developed pulmonary toxicity. Subsequently bleomycin was deleted from this regimen, and additional 26 patients were treated at the maximum tolerated dose (1.2 mg/kg of brentuximab vedotin). Despite removing bleomycin from the treatment regimen the response rate remained high, with 92% achieving complete remission at the end of 6 cycles. Remarkably, no patient developed pulmonary toxicity. A multicenter randomized study is currently enrolling patients with advanced-stage HL comparing standard ABVD therapy with brentuximab vedotin + AVD. In a different approach, the German Hodgkin Lymphoma Study Group is conducting a clinical trial incorporating brentuximab vedotin with a modified eBEACOPP regimen (clinicaltrials.gov number: NCT01569204). The results of this trial should become available in the near future.

SUMMARY

After more than 3 decades since the discovery of the CD30 molecule on the HRS cells of the in vitro cell line L428, therapeutic targeting of CD30 has become a reality.[20] In fact, brentuximab vedotin is one of the most effective single agents in patients with relapsed HL (Fig. 1). Randomized clinical trials incorporating brentuximab vedotin in

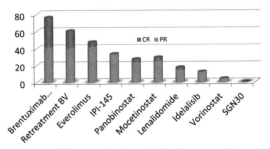

Fig. 1. Single-agent activity of brentuximab vedotin in comparison with other investigational agents in patients with relapsed Hodgkin lymphoma. CR, complete remission; PR, partial remission.

front-line, pretransplant, and posttransplant regimens are under way. Additional studies are addressing the potential value of brentuximab vedotin in early-stage disease with or without radiation therapy. Collaborative efforts among investigators and active participation of patients in these high-priority clinical trials will be required to accelerate progress, and could change the standard of care.

REFERENCES

1. Younes A. CD30-targeted antibody therapy. Curr Opin Oncol 2011;23(6):587–93.
2. Younes A, Kadin ME. Emerging applications of the tumor necrosis factor family of ligands and receptors in cancer therapy. J Clin Oncol 2003;21(18):3526–34.
3. Durkop H, Latza U, Hummel M, et al. Molecular cloning and expression of a new member of the nerve growth factor receptor family that is characteristic for Hodgkin's disease. Cell 1992;68(3):421–7.
4. Pizzolo G, Vinante F, Morosato L, et al. High serum level of the soluble form of CD30 molecule in the early phase of HIV-1 infection as an independent predictor of progression to AIDS. AIDS 1994;8(6):741–5.
5. Fattovich G, Vinante F, Giustina G, et al. Serum levels of soluble CD30 in chronic hepatitis B virus infection. Clin Exp Immunol 1996;103(1):105–10.
6. Giacomelli R, Cipriani P, Lattanzio R, et al. Circulating levels of soluble CD30 are increased in patients with systemic sclerosis (SSc) and correlate with serological and clinical features of the disease. Clin Exp Immunol 1997;108(1):42–6.
7. Bartlett NL, Younes A, Carabasi MH, et al. A phase 1 multidose study of SGN-30 immunotherapy in patients with refractory or recurrent CD30+ hematologic malignancies. Blood 2008;111(4):1848–54.
8. Ansell SM, Horwitz SM, Engert A, et al. Phase I/II study of an anti-CD30 monoclonal antibody (MDX-060) in Hodgkin's lymphoma and anaplastic large-cell lymphoma. J Clin Oncol 2007;25(19):2764–9.
9. Younes A. Beyond chemotherapy: new agents for targeted treatment of lymphoma. Nat Rev Clin Oncol 2011;8(2):85–96.
10. Younes A, Yasothan U, Kirkpatrick P. Brentuximab vedotin. Nat Rev Drug Discov 2012;11(1):19–20.
11. Katz J, Janik JE, Younes A. Brentuximab vedotin (SGN-35). Clin Cancer Res 2011;17(20):6428–36.
12. Okeley NM, Miyamoto JB, Zhang X, et al. Intracellular activation of SGN-35, a potent anti-CD30 antibody-drug conjugate. Clin Cancer Res 2010;16(3):888–97.
13. Younes A, Bartlett NL, Leonard JP, et al. Brentuximab vedotin (SGN-35) for relapsed CD30-positive lymphomas. N Engl J Med 2010;363(19):1812–21.
14. Fanale MA, Forero-Torres A, Rosenblatt JD, et al. A phase I weekly dosing study of brentuximab vedotin in patients with relapsed/refractory CD30-positive hematologic malignancies. Clin Cancer Res 2012;18(1):248–55.
15. Younes A, Gopal AK, Smith SE, et al. Results of a pivotal phase II study of brentuximab vedotin for patients with relapsed or refractory Hodgkin's lymphoma. J Clin Oncol 2012;30(18):2183–9.
16. Bartlett NL, Niedzwiecki D, Johnson JL, et al. Gemcitabine, vinorelbine, and pegylated liposomal doxorubicin (GVD), a salvage regimen in relapsed Hodgkin's lymphoma: CALGB 59804. Ann Oncol 2007;18(6):1071–9.
17. Willems PJ. Dynamic mutations hit double figures. Nat Genet 1994;8(3):213–5.
18. Marwick C. No obvious reason for HBV double hit. JAMA 1983;250(1):20.
19. Campbell R. Childhood cancer: the 'double hit' disease. Nurs Mirror 1980;151(9):ii–viii.

20. Schwab U, Stein H, Gerdes J, et al. Production of a monoclonal antibody specific for Hodgkin and Sternberg-Reed cells of Hodgkin's disease and a subset of normal lymphoid cells. Nature 1982;299(5878):65–7.
21. Chen RW, Gopal AK, Smith SE, et al. Results from a pivotal phase II study of brentuximab vedotin (SGN-35) in patients with relapsed or refractory Hodgkin lymphoma (HL). ASCO Meeting Abstracts 2011;29(15 Suppl):8031.

Combination Chemoradiotherapy in Early Hodgkin Lymphoma

Marc P.E. André, MD

KEYWORDS

- Chemotherapy • Radiotherapy • Second malignancies
- Fluorodeoxyglucose positron emission tomography

KEY POINTS

- Combined modality treatment is standard of care in localized Hodgkin lymphoma (HL) and results in an excellent cure rate but with an excess of late toxicities related to radiotherapy.
- Most of the localized patients can be cured with chemotherapy (CT) alone, but omitting radiotherapy, even in highly selected interim fluorodeoxyglucose positron emission tomography–negative patients, reduces tumor control and induces more relapse, some of them, although not all, being rescued with high-dose CT and autologous stem cell transplantation.
- The challenge is to evaluate if this excess of relapse equals or exceeds the rate of late serious effect.
- It is our goal to move toward this more individualized treatment and, possibly one day, the treatment of patients with HL will use newer drugs and be decided according to individual characteristics.

INTRODUCTION
Decades of Successes

The treatment of patients with Hodgkin lymphoma (HL) is one of the major success stories in oncology, and 70% to 90% of patients are cured of their lymphoma, depending on clinical stage and risk factors. Radiotherapy (RT) was used to cure patients with HL very early after its discovery, but more successes came in the 1960s for early-stage diseases IA and IIA with the use of extended field RT techniques to include all nodal stations above the diaphragm, such as the mantle field.[1] The addition of chemotherapy (CT) to radiation improved the cure rate, and combined modality treatment (CMT) of CT followed by localized RT became the standard treatment of patients with early-stage HL.

However, from the long follow-up that was available for these young patients, it seems that the price to pay for these successes was late toxicities, mainly secondary malignancies. CT was implicated in these secondary cancers (SCs) earlier as nitrogen

CHU Dinant Godinne, UCL Namur, 1 Avenue Thérasse, 5530 Yvoir, Belgium
E-mail address: marc.andre@uclouvain.be

Hematol Oncol Clin N Am 28 (2014) 33–47
http://dx.doi.org/10.1016/j.hoc.2013.10.010   **hemonc.theclinics.com**

mustard, vincristine, prednisone, and procarbazine (MOPP)-induced secondary leukemias. However, this CT has no longer been used since the CALGB (Cancer and Leukemia Group B) trial,[2] which showed that it was less effective and more toxic than adriamycin, bleomycin, vinblastine, and dacarbazine (ABVD). Most of the secondary malignancies are related to RT, because they occur within the field of irradiation. Other late toxicities such as cardiovascular events are related to both CT (anthracyclines) and RT. Although RT has evolved during the last decades by using lower doses and especially smaller fields, there is still a continuous trend to reducing its use (**Fig. 1**).[3] Several investigators have therefore proposed treating patients with localized HL with CT alone, because most of them can be cured with this treatment.[4] However, the price to pay for this result is an excess of relapses of the HL seen in nearly all trials. The paradigm in patients with HL is that even patients in relapse can be rescued by high-dose CT (HDCT) with autologous stem cell transplantation (ASCT) and have a chance for secondary cure.[5] The 2 proposed pathways for reaching a cure in localized HL are summarized in **Fig. 2**. Which of these pathways leads to fewer toxicities overall is the subject of considerable and sometimes furious debate[6,7] and is the subject of this article, which focuses on a combination of CT and RT in localized HL.

BACKGROUND
Treatment

RT alone is not an option
A few years after the discovery of radiographs, at the beginning of the twentieth century, HL was shown to be very sensitive to this radiation.[8] With improvements in irradiation techniques,[9] localized HL became curable with radiation therapy alone. When CT developed in the 1940s and after, HL proved to be a chemosensitive cancer.[10] The introduction of newer agents and their combination into programs, such as MOPP and ABVD by investigators, including DeVita and colleages[11] and Bonadonna and colleagues,[12] proved that HL could be cured even in advanced stages.

Several randomized trials have compared RT alone (subtotal nodal irradiation [STNI]) with CT plus RT (CMT) for patients with localized tumors (**Table 1**). The addition of CT to STNI gives even better results in terms of event-free survival (EFS), and this became the standard of care. RT alone was no longer an option. However, as the

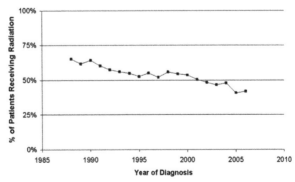

Fig. 1. Percentage of patients with HL receiving radiation between 1988 and 2006, by year of diagnosis. (*From* Koshy M, Rich SE, Mahmood U, et al. Declining use of radiotherapy in stage I and II Hodgkin's disease and its effect on survival and secondary malignancies. Int J Radiat Oncol Biol Phys 2012;82(2):621; with permission.)

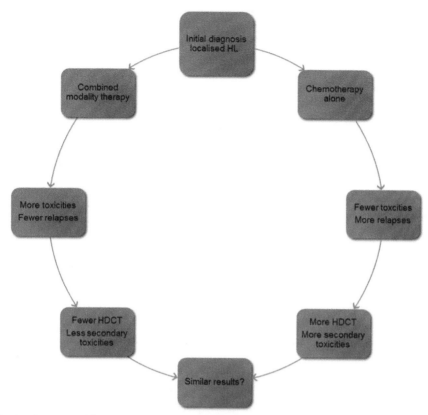

Fig. 2. The 2 possible pathways to reach definitive cure in localized HL. HDCT, high-dose chemotherapy; HL, classical Hodgkin lymphoma.

follow-up of these young patients extended, it seems that several late toxicities were associated with this success.

SCs and Late Toxicities

Evaluating the late impact of our treatments

The improved prognosis of HL has been accompanied by increased risks of SCs, cardiovascular disease, and infections. Several risk factors associated with late complications were established, which are summarized in **Table 2**. Treatments are being

Table 1
Randomized trials comparing STNI with CMT

Trial	Treatment	Number of Patients	Outcome (%)	Survival (%)
GHSG HD7[40]	A:2 ABVD + EFRT 30G	312	91	94
	B:EFRT 30G	305	75 (*P*<.001)	94
SWOG #9133[41]	A:3AV + STLI	165	94	98
	B:STLI	161	81 (*P*<.001)	96
EORTC/GELA H7 F[27]	A:6EBVP + IFRT	168	90	98
	B:STNI	168	81 (*P*<.001)	95

Table 2
Risk factors of the main complications after treatment of HL

Breast Cancer	
Evolution of risk	Increasing after 10 y
Risk factors	Female gender Age at diagnosis (<25–30 y) RT (dose, volume)
Protecting factor	Premature menopause (alkylating agents)
Lung Cancer	
Evolution of risk	More premature if the patient is older at diagnosis
Risk factors	Thoracic RT (dose dependent) Alkylating agents (dose dependent) Tobacco use
Cardiovascular	
Evolution of risk	Increase after 5–10 y
Risk factors	Thoracic RT (dose dependent) Anthracyclines (dose dependent: doxorubicin: >200–300 mg/m^2) Classic cardiovascular risks (eg, diabetes, hypertension)
Thyroid	
Evolution of risk	Continuous (peak at 3–5 y) 50% during first 10–20 y, half of them during the first 5 y
Risk factors	RT

adapted based on increased knowledge of treatment-related morbidity and mortality. However, evidence concerning late toxicities suffers from several imperfections, making interpretation of the data difficult.

First, late effects occur after long and even very long follow-up. Treatments for which long-term follow-up data are available are often no longer the standard of care. Franklin and colleagues[13] described a good example of that situation in a meta-analysis. RT as a first-line treatment strategy for stage I–III patients leads to a higher overall rate of all SC and non-Hodgkin lymphoma (NHL) than a combined modality strategy. RT alone is no longer an option, because more patients relapse compared with CMT. In the same meta-analysis, no difference in SC rates was seen between RT and CMT if follow-up times were censored at HL progression/relapse. This finding suggests that the excess SC risk after RT may be caused by the greater progression/relapse rate and therefore greater need for intensive salvage therapy.[14]

Second, the greatest source of uncertainty may be the reliability of reporting of SC. In particular, the earlier trials were not designed to provide information on SC risk; underreporting is likely. Most trials assessed their SC information as probably incomplete. Few had cross-checked with death or cancer registries. Comparison of observed SC rates with those expected from cancer registry data implied serious underreporting in a few trials. On the other hand, SC rates may be overreported, in the sense that patients without an event are more likely to be lost to follow-up. A bias in the estimation of treatment effect would result only if such reporting biases differed between treatment arms. Furthermore, some trials did not record SC.

The number of events related to late effects is small, and therefore, large cohorts of patients need to be recruited to analyze late toxicities.[15,16] In most cases, several trials are pooled or meta-analysis is performed, leading to a strong heterogeneity in the analyzed population.

CAVEATS IN INTERPRETING CLINICAL TRIALS FOR LOCALIZED HL
Absence of Evidence is Not Always Evidence of Absence

Concerning clinical trials for localized HL, several points should be emphasized to allow correct interpretation of the results.

First, patients with localized HL is generally classified in 2 categories: favorable and unfavorable. The prognostic factors used to define these 2 groups are different around the world (**Table 3**). Therefore, the results obtained for favorable patients by 1 collaborative group might not be automatically adaptable to other groups. Although some differences are minor (eg, 3 vs 4 lymph node areas), this situation is unique in lymphoma clinical research. A global consensus should certainly be reached but has not yet been obtained. Moreover, some groups like the German Hodgkin Study Group (GHSG) will include nodular lymphocyte predominant HL in their trials and others (Lymphoma Study Association [LYSA], Italian Lymphoma Foundation [FIL], European Organization for Research and Treatment of Cancer [EORTC]) will not.

Second, the primary end point of the trial should be carefully identified. This primary end point will influence the statistical design of the trial and the number of events needed to answer the question. Currently, the results reached for HL are excellent. There are, therefore, few events (relapse/refractory patients or death related to the treatment) and even fewer patients dying from the disease, because patients can be rescued by HDCT and ASCT and be cured. The primary end point of studies is therefore generally progression-free survival (PFS), and many patients are needed to answer a question in a phase 3 trial. For trials with PFS as their primary end point, the absence of difference in overall survival (OS) should not be overinterpreted. The absence of evidence for a difference cannot be translated into an evidence of absence of difference, because it generally reflects the lack of statistical power: the trial was not designed to show a difference in OS. However, a few trials will have OS as their end point. In a survival trial, the definition of an event (death) is simple. but the number of patients should be dramatically increased or the follow-up needs to be very long. With very long follow-up, additional patients will die from late toxicities and increase the number of events. The risk associated with very long follow-up is that at the time the expected number of events is reached and the data are mature, the standard of care (standard arm) may have changed and the data of the trial are no longer relevant.

Table 3				
Risk factors according to treatment groups				
		EORTC/LYSA	**GHSG**	**Canada**
RFs	A	Mediastinal mass	Mediastinal mass	
	B	Age ≥50 y	Extranodal site E	Age >40 y
	C	ESR ≥50	ESR ≥50	ESR >50 y
	D	≥4 nodal areas	≥3 nodal areas	≥3 sites
	E	B+ ESR >30		
Stage				
Favorable		I–II without RF	I–II without RF	I–II without RF
Unfavorable		I–II with RF	I–IIA with 1 or + RF	I–II with RF
			IIB with C/D without A/B	
Advanced		III–IV	IIB with A/B without C/D	III–IV
			III–IV	

Abbreviations: ESR, erythrocyte sedimentation rate; RF, risk factor.

Third, the type of trial must be considered. On one hand, in superiority trials, the experimental arm is expected to be superior to the standard arm. However, the results in localized HL are excellent, and further improvements will be small, at the price of many randomized patients. On the other hand, a reduction in the toxicity of the treatment might be the goal, and then a noninferiority trial is proposed. In this kind of trial, the experimental arm is supposed to be less toxic but nearly as effective. Usually, a slightly lower efficacy of the less toxic experimental treatment has to be accepted. The bigger the tolerated difference, the lower the number of patients needed. However, it is difficult to precisely define what is an acceptable difference with a previous standard. Would we allow a 15% difference in the PFS because we know that a lot of patients can be rescued by HDCT and ASCT? Or will we accept only 5%, because we do not want to submit our patients to intensive toxic therapies? This almost philosophic debate remains controversial.

Because the number of events is small in our trials, a few unrelated events (suicide, car accident, unexplained death) might lead to differences that confuse the interpretation.

REDUCING RT
Trying to Reduce Side Effects

Reducing the size of the RT field
Dosimetric model In a study by Koh and colleagues,[17] organ-specific SC risk estimates were estimated using a dosimetric risk modeling approach. It was shown that moving from 35-Gy mantle RT to 35-Gy involved field RT (IFRT) reduces predicted excess related risk for female breast and lung cancer by approximately 65%, and for male lung cancer by approximately 35%.

Retrospective study It is expected that the reduction of RT fields will reduce the secondary malignancies. This reduction has not yet been shown in randomized trials. However, in a retrospective study on breast cancer after HL treatment, it was shown that mantle field irradiation (involving the axillary, mediastinal, and neck nodes) was associated with a 2.7-fold increased risk (95% confidence interval [CI], 1.1–6.9) compared with similarly dosed (36–44 Gy) mediastinal irradiation alone.[18] Among patients treated with mantle field irradiation (without pelvic RT), the incidence of breast cancer was 8 times higher than in the general population (standardized incidence ratio [SIR], 8.2; 95% CI, 6.6–10.1) compared with 3.7 (SIR, 3.7; 95% CI, 1.2–8.7) for those receiving mediastinal IFRT (without pelvic RT). This type of effect has not yet been shown for other cancers, especially lung cancer.

Randomized trials
HD8 A total of 1204 patients were randomized to 4 cycles of CT followed by either 30-Gy extended field RT (EFRT) or 30-Gy IFRT; 532 patients in each treatment arm were eligible. At 10 years, no arm differences were revealed with respect to freedom from treatment failure (FFTF) (79.8% vs 79.7%), PFS (79.8% vs 80.0%), and OS (86.4% vs 87.3%). Noninferiority of IFRT was shown for the primary end point FFTF (95% CI for hazard ratio [HR] 0.72–1.25). Moreover, elderly patients had a poorer outcome when treated with EFRT. At the time of publication, 15.0% of patients in the EFRT arm and 12.2% in the IFRT arm had died, mostly because of secondary malignancies (5.3% vs 3.4%) or HL (3.2% vs 3.4%). After EFRT, there were more secondary malignancies overall (58 vs 45), especially acute myeloid leukemias (11 vs 4). RT intensity reduction to IFRT did not result in poorer long-term outcome but was associated with less acute toxicity and might be associated with fewer secondary malignancies.

H8-U In this trial, 3 regimens were compared: 6 cycles of mustargen, oncovin, pro-carbazine, prednisone (MOPP) and adriamycin, bleomycin, vinblastine (ABV) plus IFRT (reference group), 4 cycles of MOPP-ABV plus IFRT, and 4 cycles of MOPP-ABV plus subtotal nodal RT.[19] The estimated 5-year EFS rates were similar in the 3 treatment groups: 84%, 88%, and 87%, respectively. The 10-year OS estimates were 88%, 85%, and 84%.

Milan #9005 The trial compared 4 ABVD plus IFRT versus 4 ABVD versus STNI in stage IA, IB, and IIA patients.[20] The 12-year freedom from progression rates were 93% after ABVD and STNI, and 94% after ABVD and IFRT, whereas the figures for OS were 96% and 94%, respectively.

HD94 A total of 210 patients with Hodgkin disease, at clinical stage II with risk fac-tors and III without risk factors received 4 ABVD.[21] Patients who achieved complete response (CR) or partial response (PR) were randomized to the IFRT or EFRT. OS was 98% and 96%, respectively, in the EFRT and IFRT arms and recurrence-free sur-vival (RFS) was 94% and 91%, respectively, in the EFRT and IFRT arms.

Recently, clinical trials have used even more limited fields, referred to as involved node RT (INRT). The concept of INRT was developed initially in the EORTC-LYSA-FIL[22] and has been adopted by other clinical trials groups. INRT is attractive because the irradiated volume is less, and a smaller volume of radiation treatment must be associated with less risk for late effects. Preliminary data confirming this concept have been published.[23] Whereas the EORTC/LYSA/FIL have already adopted INRT in their clinical trials, the GHSG has chosen to test the concept against the IFRT stan-dard. In the GHSG HD17 trial, patients who are treated with combined modality therapy are randomized to treatment with IFRT or, depending on the result of fluoro-deoxyglucose (FDG) positron emission tomography (PET) after 4 cycles of CT, either INRT (PET positive) or no further treatment (NFT) (PET negative).

Reducing the dose of RT
Radiation dose was identified as 1 relevant risk factor associated with the risk of sec-ondary malignancies. For breast,[24] lung,[25] and thyroid cancer, there is a direct rela-tionship between dose and risk. Radiation dose is also associated with the risk of cardiovascular disease and lung fibrosis. Therefore, there is a strong need for pro-spective clinical studies on treatment with reduced intensity of RT.

The HD10 trial In this trial, 1370 patients with newly diagnosed early-stage HL with a favorable prognosis received 2 or 4 ABVD and were randomized to either 30 Gy or 20 Gy IFRT (factorial design).[26] The primary end point was FFTF. When the doses of RT (20-Gy and 30-Gy) were compared, the rate of FFTF at 5 years was 93.4% (95% CI, 91.0–95.2) in the 30-Gy group and 92.9% (95% CI, 90.4–94.8) in the 20-Gy group. The HR for treatment failure with 20 Gy compared with 30 Gy was 1.00 (95% CI, 0.68–1.47). Adverse events and acute toxic effects of treatment were most common in the patients who received 4 cycles of ABVD and 30 Gy of radiation therapy.

The H9F trial The aim of the H9F trial was to assess whether IFRT to a lower dose than 30 to 36 Gy or no RT after CT could be used without compromising the high rate of disease control in patients with early-stage HL without risk factors.[27] After a median follow-up of 33 months, the results of the trial showed that in patients in CR after 6 cy-cles of epirubicin, bleomycin, vinblastine and prednisone (EBVP), 20 Gy of IFRT is equivalent to 36 Gy of IFRT with a 4-year EFS rate of 87% in the 36-Gy arm and 84% in the 20-Gy arm. In contrast, a treatment avoiding RT provides significantly worse results both in terms of relapse-free survival and EFS (4-year EFS: 70% in the 0-Gy arm [*P*<.001]); premature closure of recruitment in this group was necessary. However, the 4-year OS was 98% in all 3 arms.

It appeared from these 2 trials than both the amount of CT and the dose or RT can be reduced without affecting the quality of the results in patients with favorable prognostic factors. This statement cannot be applied to localized patients with unfavorable risk factors. In the HD11 trial,[28] 1395 patients were randomized first for CT (ABVD vs bleomycin, etoposide, doxorubicin, cyclophosphamide, vincristine, procarbazine, prednisone [BEACOPP] baseline) and then for RT (30 Gy vs 20 Gy). There was no difference between BEACOPP baseline and ABVD when followed by 30-Gy IFRT. After 4 cycles of BEACOPP baseline, 20 Gy was not inferior to 30 Gy, whereas inferiority of 20 Gy cannot be excluded after 4 cycles of ABVD.

CT ALONE
The Ultimate Reduction of Radiotherapy

Even with modern reduction of the dose and RT, all side effects will probably not be eliminated. Therefore, omission of RT would be the safest way to go as far as late toxicities are concerned. CT alone was performed in countries where RT was not available, with excellent results. Several trials then compared CT alone with CMT, and a meta-analysis was recently completed of these trials.[29] Five randomized controlled trials involving 1245 patients were included (**Table 4**). The HR was 0.41 (95% CI 0.25–0.66) for tumor control and 0.40 (95% CI 0.27–0.59) for OS for patients receiving CMT compared with CT alone. CR rates were similar between treatment groups. In sensitivity analyses, another 6 trials were included that did not fulfill the inclusion criteria of the meta-analysis but were considered relevant to the topic. These trials underlined the results of the main analysis. The conclusion is that adding RT to CT improves tumor control and OS in patients with early-stage HL. However, most of these trials, including most that contributed to the meta-analysis, incorporated CT regimens, such as EBVP, now known to be inferior to ABVD, and thus do not properly inform current decision making.

Table 4
Trials included in the meta-analysis[29] comparing CMT and CT alone

Trial	Inclusion Criteria	Number of Patients	Treatment	Median Follow-Up y (Range)
Mexico B2H031[42]	CSI-II	99 10	6 ABVD 6 ABVD + MFRT	11.4 (6.3–16.5)
CALGB 7751[43]	PSI-II	18 19	6 CVPP 6 CVPP + IFRT	2 (not reported)
EORTC-GELA H9F[27]	CSI-II Favorable	130 448	6 EBVP 6 EBVP + IFRT	4.3 (1.3–6.8)
GATLA-9-H-77[44]	CSI-II Favorable and unfavorable	142 135	6 CVPP 6 CVPP + IFRT	4 (not reported)
MSCKK 90–44[45]	CSI-IIIA	76 76	6 ABVD 6 ABVD + IFRT/EFRT	5.6 (0.1–10.4)

Abbreviations: CS I-II, clinical stage I-II; PS I-II, pathological stage I-II; MFRT, mantle field radiotherapy.
From Herbst C, Rehan FA, Skoetz N, et al. Chemotherapy alone versus chemotherapy plus radiotherapy for early stage Hodgkin lymphoma. Cochrane Database Syst Rev 2011;(2):CD007110; with permission.

More recently, a study from the SEER (Surveillance Epidemiology and End Results) database, which included patients who were 20 years and older who had been diagnosed from 1988 to 2006 with stage I or II HD, was published.[3] A total of 12,247 patients were selected and 51.5% received RT. In the period 1988 to 1991, 62.9% received RT, whereas in 2004 to 2006, only 43.7% received RT (P<.001). Over this period (1988–2006), the use of radiation in stage I and II HL has decreased by more than 20% (see **Fig. 1**). The 5-year OS was 76% for patients who did not receive RT and 87% for those who did receive RT (P<.001). The HR adjusted for other variables in regression model showed that patients who did not receive RT (HR, 1.72; 95% CI, 1.72–2.02) were associated with significantly worse survival when compared with patients who received RT. The actuarial rate of developing a second malignancy was 14.6% versus 15.0% at 15 years for patients who received RT versus those with no RT (P = .089). The study has all the limitations of a registry study: information on bulky mediastinum, type of CT regimen, and doses and field of RT used are missing. However, it is a good picture of what is happening in the general population outside selected patients from the clinical trials.

The largest trial testing CT alone is the NCIC CTG HD.6 trial.[4] In the favorable cohort, there was no significant difference in EFS and OS between treatment with ABVD or STNI. In the unfavorable cohort, the rate of OS was higher among patients in the ABVD-only group than among the patients in the radiation therapy group who received subtotal nodal radiation therapy plus ABVD (12-year estimates, 92% vs 81%; P = .04), whereas the rate of freedom from disease progression was lower in the ABVD-only group (12-year estimates, 86% vs 94%; P = .006). Several criticisms arose from this study. First, the radiation used (EFRT) is outdated. IFRT and also INRT are used, and the size of the RT field is important for SCs. Second, the dose used (35 cGy) is also outdated, and the dose, also related to SC risk, used is reduced to 30 and even 20 cGy for patients with a favorable profile. Third, in this trial, it is unclear whether the secondary malignancies occurred within RT. Five deaths occurred from miscellaneous causes, all in the RT arm, which largely contributes to the excess of death in the RT arm.

INTERIM FDG-PET SCAN
Tailoring the Treatment?

Introduction

Since its introduction to the diagnostic armamentarium, FDG-PET, integrated with a computed tomography scan, has rapidly evolved to become an essential diagnostic tool in HL staging, restaging, and response evaluation. Consequently, FDG-PET is now considered an integral part of HL management. Its usefulness at diagnosis and at the end of treatment is now clearly defined.

At diagnosis, FDG-PET upstages and downstages some patients, leading to 15% to 20% and 5% to 15% changes in stage and treatment, respectively.[30] However, the impact of these treatment modifications has never been evaluated prospectively.

End-of-therapy response assessment was one of the first clinical applications of FDG-PET imaging in oncology, and several reports were published emphasizing its usefulness. In a recent meta-analysis,[31] the pooled sensitivity and specificity of PET in distinguishing between different treatment outcomes in HL was 84%. In the HD15 trial of the GHSG, consolidation RT was selectively administered to patients with advanced stage HL who had a PET-positive residual mass of more than 2.5 cm at the end of CT, using 3 different BEACOPP regimens. The 4-year PFS of irradiated and nonirradiated patients was 86.2% and 92.6%, respectively (P = .022).

The negative predictive value of end-therapy PET was 94%.[32] These data suggest that RT can be safely omitted in patients with advanced stage HL who are PET negative after BEACOPP$_{escalated}$ treatment, whereas the decision to irradiate a PET-positive lesion should be made with the awareness of false-positive results as well as the lack of success in those with radiation-resistant disease.

Interim FDG-PET
An FDG-PET performed after a few cycles of CT, generally 2, seems also to be a useful tool for final outcome both for localized and advanced HL. After 2 cycles of ABVD, 75%–85% of localized HL can achieve PET negativity and have an excellent outcome.[33] However, the timing of the interim FDG-PET (iPET) should be correctly scheduled to avoid false-negative results because of tumor stunning.

To harmonize interpretations and avoid uncertainties associated with minimal residual uptake, standardization was proposed. The first standardization initiative was proposed in 2007 by the imaging subcommittee of the International Harmonization Project in lymphoma, which provided criteria for a positive FDG-PET scan after completion of therapy.[34] According to these criteria, uptake greater than that in the mediastinal blood pool in residual masses larger than 2 cm is considered positive for residual lymphoma. More recently, to better address several concerns, at a consensus meeting in Deauville, the 5-point scale system was proposed to allow for a continuous reading scheme suitable for different positivity thresholds to adjust for the intended treatment end points (**Table 5**)[35] and to minimize false-positive results by using a higher threshold applying liver uptake as the reference site. The reproducibility of these Deauville criteria was recently validated in a retrospective validation study of 260 patients with advanced stage HL.[33]

Clinical studies
Although it has been shown that the result of an iPET is predictive of treatment outcome, it remains to be proved that iPET can be used as a tool to modulate treatment intensity and personalize the treatment. Several trials have been run or are ongoing to explore the feasibility of avoiding RT for early-stage patients who are iPET negative (**Table 6**). The results of 2 of these trials were recently presented at the American Society of Hematology meeting and are further discussed.

RAPID trial Patients received 3 cycles ABVD followed by centrally reviewed FDG-PET.[36] If the PET was reported negative, patients were randomized between IFRT and NFT. A total of 602 patients with newly diagnosed stages IA/IIA HL were

Table 5 The Deauville 5-point scale for interim PET evaluation	
Score	**Description**
1	No uptake
2	Uptake ≤ mediastinum
3	Uptake > mediastinum but ≤ liver
4	Moderately increased uptake > liver
5	Markedly increased uptake > liver or new lesions related to lymphoma
X	New areas of uptake unlikely to be related to lymphoma

Data from Meignan M, Gallamini A, Haioun C, et al. Report on the Second International Workshop on interim positron emission tomography in lymphoma held in Menton, France, 8–9 April 2010. Leuk Lymphoma 2010;51(12):2177.

Table 6
Clinical trials on interim PET in localized HL

Sponsor	Code	Stage	Target Accrual
NHSFT	RAPID	Early IA-IIA	600
EORTC/LYSA/FIL	H10	Early favorable and unfavorable	1975
GHSG	HD16	Early favorable	1100
GHSG	HD17	Early unfavorable	1100
CALGB	50,801	Early bulky	123
CALGB	50,604	Early nonbulky	149
ECOG	2410	Early bulky	200

registered, and after 3 cycles of ABVD, 571 patients had a PET, of whom 426 (74.6%) were classified as PET negative. A total of 420 PET-negative patients were randomized to receive IFRT (n = 209) or NFT (n = 211). After a median follow-up of 45.7 months from randomization, in the IFRT arm of the randomized PET-negative population, 194 patients were alive and progression-free, 9 had progressed, and 6 had died. In the NFT arm, 190 patients were alive and progression-free, 20 had progressed, and 1 had died. The 3-year PFS was 93.8% IFRT versus 90.7% NFT (risk difference, 2.9%; 95% CI, 10.7%–1.4%; the lower limit marginally exceeds the maximum allowable difference of –7%). These results show that in early-stage HL, patients with a negative PET after 3 cycles of ABVD have an excellent prognosis without any further treatment. A per-protocol analysis was carried out on 392 PET-negative patients who received the assigned treatment; the 3-year PFS was 97% for IFRT and 90.7% for NFT (P = .03) in favor of the RT arm.

H10 trial Patients with stage I and II supradiaphragmatic HL, between 15 and 70 years old, were included in the study and stratified according to LYSA/EORTC criteria.[22] The schema of the study is described in **Fig. 3**. At the time of the prospectively planned interim analysis, 1137 patients were included, with a median follow-up of 1.1 years, with sufficient events to allow for the planned interim analysis. In the F early PET-negative group, 188 patients were included in the standard arm, and 193 in the experimental arm. Ten events occurred: 1 in the standard arm and 9 in the experimental arm. All these events were progressions or relapses. Based on the information fraction (10 of the 26 events required for the final analysis) and the resulting 1-sided

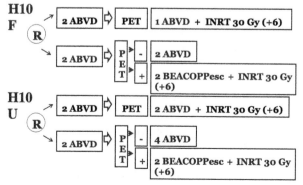

Fig. 3. EORTC/LYSA/FIL H10 (number 20051) study design.

significance level to perform the statistical test (0.102), futility was declared (P value = .017<.102). The estimated HR was 9.36 (79.6% CI, 2.45–35.73). PFS rates at 1 year were 100.0% and 94.9% in the standard and experimental arms, respectively. In the U early PET-negative group, 251 patients were included in the standard arm and 268 in the experimental arm. A total of 23 events occurred in this group: 7 in the standard arm and 16 in the experimental arm. One patient died because of bleomycin toxicity without signs of progression; all remaining events were progressions or relapses. Based on the information fraction (23 of the 63 events required for the final analysis) and the resulting 1-sided significance level to perform the statistical test (0.098), futility was declared (P value = .026<.098). The estimated HR was 2.42 (80.4% CI, 1.35–4.36). PFS rates at 1 year were 97.3% and 94.7% in the standard and experimental arms, respectively. The interim analysis for the early PET-positive group gave no reason for stopping this part of the trial. Final accrual was reached in June 2011 with 1950 patients included. The planned futility IA of the H10 trial shows that the risk of early relapse in nonirradiated patients with stage I–II HL was significantly higher than in patients treated with the standard combined modality, even in this selected group of patients with an early negative PET. Consequently, accrual was stopped for this part of the trial.

iPET conclusion It is clear from several studies that patients with localized HL can be cured with CT alone and that only a few them benefit from RT. The expectation was that interim PET would identify patients who do not need RT and are equally well cured with CT alone. In the 2 completed randomized trials that are available, it seems that the experimental arms (without RT) tend to have a poorer PFS than CMT. Moreover, these results were observed in clinical trials with a conservative definition of PET negativity and central review of the images. These specific conditions are not available in routine clinical practice, and the results of these trials cannot be simply implemented into daily practice.[37] Therefore, it should be clearly emphasized that the place of interim PET in treatment adaptation needs longer follow-up and results of additional randomized studies such as the GHSG trials HD16 and HD17.

SUMMARY
Not One Size Fits All

CMT is the standard of care in localized HL[38] and results in an excellent cure rate but with an excess of late toxicities related to RT. Most of the localized patients can be cured with CT alone, but omitting RT, even in highly selected iPET-negative patients, reduces tumor control and induces more relapse, some of them, although not all, being rescued with HDCT and ASCT. The challenge will be to evaluate if this excess of relapse will equal or exceed the rate of late serious effects. It is our goal to move toward this more individualized treatment and, possibly one day, the treatment of patients with HL will use newer drugs[39] and be decided according to individual characteristics.

REFERENCES

1. Kaplan HS, Rosenberg SA. Extended-field radical radiotherapy in advanced Hodgkin's disease: short-term results of 2 randomized clinical trials. Cancer Res 1966;26(6):1268–72.
2. Canellos GP, Anderson JR, Propert KJ, et al. Chemotherapy of advanced Hodgkin's disease with MOPP, ABVD, or MOPP alternating with ABVD. N Engl J Med 1992;327(21):1478–84.

3. Koshy M, Rich SE, Mahmood U, et al. Declining use of radiotherapy in stage I and II Hodgkin's disease and its effect on survival and secondary malignancies. Int J Radiat Oncol Biol Phys 2012;82(2):619–25.
4. Meyer RM, Gospodarowicz MK, Connors JM, et al. ABVD alone versus radiation-based therapy in limited-stage Hodgkin's lymphoma. N Engl J Med 2012;366(5):399–408.
5. Schmitz N, Pfistner B, Sextro M, et al. Aggressive conventional chemotherapy compared with high-dose chemotherapy with autologous haemopoietic stem-cell transplantation for relapsed chemosensitive Hodgkin's disease: a randomised trial. Lancet 2002;359(9323):2065–71.
6. Yahalom J. Don't throw out the baby with the bathwater: on optimizing cure and reducing toxicity in Hodgkin's lymphoma. J Clin Oncol 2006;24(4):544–8.
7. Longo DL. Radiation therapy in Hodgkin disease: why risk a Pyrrhic victory? J Natl Cancer Inst 2005;97(19):1394–5.
8. Pusey W. Cases of sarcoma and of Hodgkin's disease treated by exposure to X-rays: a preliminary report. JAMA 1902;38:166–9.
9. Kaplan H. The radical radiotherapy of regionally localized Hodgkin's disease. Radiology 1962;78:553–61.
10. Goodman LS, Wintrobe MM, Dameshek W, et al. Nitrogen mustard therapy: use of methyl-bis (beta-chloroethyl) amine hydrochloride and tris (beta-chloroethyl) amine hydrochloride for Hodgkin's disease, lymphosarcoma, leukemia and certain allied and miscellaneous disorders. J Am Med Assoc 1946;132:126–32.
11. Devita VT Jr, Serpick AA, Carbone PP. Combination chemotherapy in the treatment of advanced Hodgkin's disease. Ann Intern Med 1970;73(6):881–95.
12. Bonadonna G, Zucali R, Monfardini S, et al. Combination chemotherapy of Hodgkin's disease with adriamycin, bleomycin, vinblastine, and imidazole carboxamide versus MOPP. Cancer 1975;36(1):252–9.
13. Franklin J, Pluetschow A, Paus M, et al. Second malignancy risk associated with treatment of Hodgkin's lymphoma: meta-analysis of the randomised trials. Ann Oncol 2006;17(12):1749–60.
14. Andre M, Henry-Amar M, Blaise D, et al. Treatment-related deaths and second cancer risk after autologous stem-cell transplantation for Hodgkin's disease. Blood 1998;92(6):1933–40.
15. Favier O, Heutte N, Stamatoullas-Bastard A, et al. Survival after Hodgkin lymphoma: causes of death and excess mortality in patients treated in 8 consecutive trials. Cancer 2009;115(8):1680–91.
16. Specht L, Gray RG, Clarke MJ, et al. Influence of more extensive radiotherapy and adjuvant chemotherapy on long-term outcome of early-stage Hodgkin's disease: a meta-analysis of 23 randomized trials involving 3,888 patients. International Hodgkin's Disease Collaborative Group. J Clin Oncol 1998;16(3):830–43.
17. Koh ES, Tran TH, Heydarian M, et al. A comparison of mantle versus involved-field radiotherapy for Hodgkin's lymphoma: reduction in normal tissue dose and second cancer risk. Radiat Oncol 2007;2:13.
18. De Bruin ML, Sparidans J, van't Veer MB, et al. Breast cancer risk in female survivors of Hodgkin's lymphoma: lower risk after smaller radiation volumes. J Clin Oncol 2009;27(26):4239–46.
19. Ferme C, Eghbali H, Meerwaldt JH, et al. Chemotherapy plus involved-field radiation in early-stage Hodgkin's disease. N Engl J Med 2007;357(19):1916–27.
20. Bonadonna G, Bonfante V, Viviani S, et al. ABVD plus subtotal nodal versus involved-field radiotherapy in early-stage Hodgkin's disease: long-term results. J Clin Oncol 2004;22(14):2835–41.

21. Anselmo AP, Cavalieri E, Osti FM, et al. Intermediate stage Hodgkin's disease: preliminary results on 210 patients treated with four ABVD chemotherapy cycles plus extended versus involved field radiotherapy. Anticancer Res 2004;24(6): 4045–50.
22. André M, Reman O, Federico M, et al. Interim Analysis of the randomized EORTC/LYSA/FIL Intergroup H10 trial on early PET-scan driven treatment adaptation in stage I/II Hodgkin lymphoma. Blood 2012;120:#549.
23. Maraldo MV, Aznar MC, Vogelius IR, et al. Involved node radiation therapy: an effective alternative in early-stage Hodgkin lymphoma. Int J Radiat Oncol Biol Phys 2013;85(4):1057–65.
24. Travis LB, Hill DA, Dores GM, et al. Breast cancer following radiotherapy and chemotherapy among young women with Hodgkin disease. JAMA 2003;290(4): 465–75.
25. Travis LB, Gospodarowicz M, Curtis RE, et al. Lung cancer following chemotherapy and radiotherapy for Hodgkin's disease. J Natl Cancer Inst 2002;94(3):182–92.
26. Engert A, Plutschow A, Eich HT, et al. Reduced treatment intensity in patients with early-stage Hodgkin's lymphoma. N Engl J Med 2010;363(7):640–52.
27. Thomas J, Fermé C, Noordijk EM, et al. Results of the EORTC-GELA H9 randomized trials: the H9-F trial (comparing 3 radiation dose levels) and H9-U trial (comparing 3 chemotherapy schemes) in patients with favorable or unfavorable early stage Hodgkin's lymphoma (HL). Haematologica 2007;92(Suppl 5):27.
28. Eich HT, Diehl V, Gorgen H, et al. Intensified chemotherapy and dose-reduced involved-field radiotherapy in patients with early unfavorable Hodgkin's lymphoma: final analysis of the German Hodgkin Study Group HD11 trial. J Clin Oncol 2010;28(27):4199–206.
29. Herbst C, Rehan FA, Skoetz N, et al. Chemotherapy alone versus chemotherapy plus radiotherapy for early stage Hodgkin lymphoma. Cochrane Database Syst Rev 2011;(2):CD007110.
30. Seam P, Juweid ME, Cheson BD. The role of FDG-PET scans in patients with lymphoma. Blood 2007;110(10):3507–16.
31. Terasawa T, Nihashi T, Hotta T, et al. 18F-FDG PET for posttherapy assessment of Hodgkin's disease and aggressive non-Hodgkin's lymphoma: a systematic review. J Nucl Med 2008;49(1):13–21.
32. Engert A, Haverkamp H, Kobe C, et al. Reduced-intensity chemotherapy and PET-guided radiotherapy in patients with advanced stage Hodgkin's lymphoma (HD15 trial): a randomised, open-label, phase 3 non-inferiority trial. Lancet 2012;379(9828):1791–9.
33. Biggi A, Gallamini A, Chauvie S, et al. International validation study for interim PET in ABVD-treated, advanced-stage Hodgkin lymphoma: interpretation criteria and concordance rate among reviewers. J Nucl Med 2013;54(5):683–90.
34. Juweid ME, Stroobants S, Hoekstra OS, et al. Use of positron emission tomography for response assessment of lymphoma: consensus of the Imaging Subcommittee of International Harmonization Project in Lymphoma. J Clin Oncol 2007; 25(5):571–8.
35. Meignan M, Gallamini A, Haioun C, et al. Report on the Second International Workshop on interim positron emission tomography in lymphoma held in Menton, France, 8–9 April 2010. Leuk Lymphoma 2010;51(12):2171–80.
36. Radford J, Barrington S, Counsell N, et al. Involved field radiotherapy versus no further treatment in patients with clinical stages IA and IIA Hodgkin lymphoma and a 'Negative' PET scan after 3 cycles ABVD. Results of the UK NCRI RAPID Trial. Blood 2012;120:#547.

37. Radford J. Treatment for early-stage Hodgkin lymphoma: has radiotherapy had its day? J Clin Oncol 2012;30(31):3783–5.
38. Eichenauer DA, Engert A, Dreyling M. Hodgkin's lymphoma: ESMO clinical practice guidelines for diagnosis, treatment and follow-up. Ann Oncol 2011;22(Suppl 6):vi55–8.
39. Younes A, Gopal AK, Smith SE, et al. Results of a pivotal phase II study of brentuximab vedotin for patients with relapsed or refractory Hodgkin's lymphoma. J Clin Oncol 2012;30(18):2183–9.
40. Engert A, Franklin J, Eich HT, et al. Two cycles of doxorubicin, bleomycin, vinblastine, and dacarbazine plus extended-field radiotherapy is superior to radiotherapy alone in early favorable Hodgkin's lymphoma: final results of the GHSG HD7 trial. J Clin Oncol 2007;25(23):3495–502.
41. Press OW, LeBlanc M, Lichter AS, et al. Phase III randomized Intergroup trial of subtotal lymphoid irradiation versus doxorubicin, vinblastine, and subtotal lymphoid irradiation for stage IA to IIA Hodgkin's disease. J Clin Oncol 2001; 19(22):4238–44.
42. Aviles A, Delgado S. A prospective clinical trial comparing chemotherapy, radiotherapy and combined therapy in the treatment of early stage Hodgkin's disease with bulky disease. Clin Lab Haematol 1998;20(2):95–9.
43. Bloomfield CD, Pajak TF, Glicksman AS, et al. Chemotherapy and combined modality therapy for Hodgkin's disease: a progress report on Cancer and Leukemia Group B studies. Cancer Treat Rep 1982;66(4):835–46.
44. Pavlovsky S, Maschio M, Santarelli MT, et al. Randomized trial of chemotherapy versus chemotherapy plus radiotherapy for stage I-II Hodgkin's disease. J Natl Cancer Inst 1988;80(18):1466–73.
45. Straus DJ, Portlock CS, Qin J, et al. Results of a prospective randomized clinical trial of doxorubicin, bleomycin, vinblastine, and dacarbazine (ABVD) followed by radiation therapy (RT) versus ABVD alone for stages I, II, and IIIA nonbulky Hodgkin disease. Blood 2004;104(12):3483–9.

Balancing Risks and Benefits of Therapy for Patients with Favorable-Risk Limited-Stage Hodgkin Lymphoma

The Role of Doxorubicin, Bleomycin, Vinblastine, and Dacarbazine Chemotherapy Alone

Annette E. Hay, MB ChB, MRCP, FRCPath[a],
Ralph M. Meyer, MD, FRCP(C)[b],*

KEYWORDS

- Hodgkin lymphoma • Chemotherapy • Combined modality therapy
- Radiation therapy • Review

KEY POINTS

- More than 80% of patients with stage IA to IIA nonbulky Hodgkin lymphoma are cured with doxorubicin, bleomycin, vinblastine, and dacarbazine (ABVD) chemotherapy alone.
- Death after a diagnosis of Hodgkin lymphoma is more commonly caused by factors unrelated to disease progression and includes treatment-related adverse late effects.
- Follow-up into the third decade after treatment is required to properly assess overall survival after radiation therapy.
- Refinement of early response assessment using positron emission tomography–computed tomography scans may assist individualizing therapy, including defining those who may benefit most from combined modality therapy.

INTRODUCTION

Current controversies in managing patients with Hodgkin lymphoma are a result of uncertainties in balancing the best measures to eradicate the disease while minimizing the risks of long-term adverse effects that are associated with available therapies.

Disclosure statement: Dr Meyer has received consulting fees from Lilly and Celgene for roles on Data Safety Monitoring and Independent Response Assessment Committees, respectively. Dr Hay has no conflicts of interest to declare.
[a] NCIC Clinical Trials Group, Queen's University, 10 Stuart Street, Kingston, Ontario K7L 3N6, Canada; [b] Juravinski Hospital and Cancer Centre, Cancer Care Ontario, 711 Concession Street, Hamilton, Ontario L8V 1C3, Canada
* Corresponding author.
E-mail address: Ralph.Meyer@jcc.hhsc.ca

Hematol Oncol Clin N Am 28 (2014) 49–63
http://dx.doi.org/10.1016/j.hoc.2013.10.001
0889-8588/14/$ – see front matter © 2014 Elsevier Inc. All rights reserved.

For patients with localized Hodgkin lymphoma and favorable-risk features, debates relate to the relative merits of treatment with doxorubicin, bleomycin, vinblastine, and dacarbazine (ABVD) chemotherapy alone versus combining fewer cycles of this treatment with localized radiation therapy (RT); for those with advanced disease, debates center around use of ABVD versus bleomycin, etoposide, doxorubicin, cyclophosphamide, vincristine, prednisone, and procarbazine (BEACOPP). Common to both debates is realization that most clinical trials that inform practices do not directly address the morbidities and mortality that become apparent in the second and third decades after treatment and that available data about these long-term outcomes relate to previous treatment strategies that are now outdated.

Reviews describing these debates benefit from placing current perspectives onto a background of previous accomplishments in managing patients with Hodgkin lymphoma. Early in the twentieth century, the diagnosis was fatal to all but a few with accessible, localized tumors, in whom radical surgical excision afforded freedom from disease.[1,2] Pioneers in RT discovered means to control localized disease,[3–5] over time observing fewer relapses with increasing radiation fields, leading to adoption of extended-field irradiation encompassing the mantle field (axillary, mediastinal, and axillary nodes), spleen, and para-aortic region.[6,7] Simultaneously, chemotherapy evolved from single-agent nitrogen mustard[8] to combinations resulting in the possibility of cure, even for those with advanced disease.[9] Cure rates increased with coadministration of radiation and chemotherapy, termed combined modality therapy (CMT).[10] By the turn of the millennium, long-term disease control was observed in 80% to 90% of those with favorable limited-stage Hodgkin lymphoma treated with CMT, and many reports described cure rates of greater than 90%.[10–12] With long-term follow-up of young survivors, there was increasing recognition of the problem of late treatment-related toxicities, resulting in premature death, despite cure of Hodgkin lymphoma.[13] Over recent decades, strategies attempting to reduce late effects and maintain or improve disease control in newly diagnosed patients have included adoption of ABVD as the standard chemotherapy regimen because it is more effective than historical regimens and is not associated with the risks of leukemogenesis or gonadal toxicity,[14] reduction of radiation from extended to involved fields,[11] abbreviation of the number of cycles of chemotherapy as part of CMT,[15] and omission of RT by using ABVD chemotherapy alone.[16–18]

The objective of this review is to describe the rationale and context of a treatment decision to use chemotherapy alone as treatment of patients with stage IA and IIA nonbulky Hodgkin lymphoma, building on evidence presented in a recent review.[19] As described in that review, a focus of the current debate about treatment options has been the reporting of the final results of the NCIC Clinical Trials Group (NCIC CTG)–Eastern Cooperative Oncology Group (ECOG) HD.6 trial, in which patients with stage IA and IIA nonbulky Hodgkin lymphoma were randomized to receive 4 to 6 cycles of ABVD alone (the choice of 4 vs 6 cycles was based on disease-control assessment after 2 treatment cycles) or subtotal nodal radiation, given as a single modality to patients younger than 40 years who had no more than 3 nodal sites of disease and an erythrocyte sedimentation rate (ESR) of less than 50, or combined with 2 cycles of ABVD for patients not satisfying these 3 qualifying criteria.[16] The main results of this trial were that chemotherapy alone was associated with superior 12-year overall survival (94% vs 87%; hazard ratio [HR] = 0.50, 95% confidence interval [CI], 0.25–0.99; $P = .04$) but inferior disease control as assessed by 12-year freedom from disease progression (87% vs 92%; HR = 1.91, 95% CI, 0.99–3.69; $P = .05$). Superior overall survival with ABVD alone was because fewer deaths were observed attributed to causes other than Hodgkin lymphoma.

PATIENT POPULATION AND CURRENT GUIDELINES

Several bodies have used various approaches to consider evidence and reach consensus to produce practice guideline recommendations intended to assist those managing patients with favorable-risk, limited-stage Hodgkin lymphoma (**Table 1**).[20–23] Although some details differ, these bodies have generally defined this population as those with stage IA and IIA nonbulky disease. Added factors used by some have included the number of nodal sites or areas, ESR and, less commonly in selected patients, B symptoms. Our discussion is based on a population that includes all those with stage IA and IIA, nonbulky disease excepting those rare patients with these features who also have intra-abdominal disease. We have chosen these parameters because they were used as eligibility criteria in the NCIC CTG-ECOG HD.6 trial.[16,24]

Allowing for slight differences in population definition, recommendations from all 4 guideline bodies include use of CMT with 2 to 4 cycles of ABVD and involved-field RT (IFRT) with 20 to 30 Gy (variations within these ranges depend on patient specifics). In addition, one body, the National Comprehensive Cancer Network (NCCN), also includes 4 to 6 cycles of ABVD alone as an acceptable alternative, but assigns this recommendation a lower level of evidence (level 2A). Of these 4 guidelines, only the NCCN guidelines included consideration of the final analysis of the HD.6 trial, which was published in 2012 and reported 12-year outcomes.[16] The other 3 bodies published their recommendations before 2012 and considered the initial HD.6 results,

Table 1
Current treatment guidelines for patients with stage I to II Hodgkin lymphoma

Guideline Body	Patient Population	Recommended Therapy
National Comprehensive Cancer Network, 2013[20]	Stage IA–IIA favorable disease: no mediastinal bulk, peripheral disease ≤10 cm, ESR ≤50, ≤3 sites of disease	CMT (2–4 ABVD + ISRT) (category 1) or Stanford V × 8 weeks (category 2A) or ABVD alone (category 2A)
European Society for Medical Oncology, 2011[21]	Stage IA–IIA without risk factors: GHSG – large mediastinal mass, extranodal disease, increased ESR, ≥3 nodal areas; EORTC/GELA – large mediastinal mass, age ≥50 y, increased ESR, ≥4 nodal areas	2 cycles of ABVD + 20-Gy IFRT (grade A recommendation)
Italian Society of Haematology, 2009[22]	Stage I–II favorable disease: EORTC – ≤3 nodal involved areas, age <50 y, and M/T ratio <0.33, and ESR <50 without B symptoms, or ESR <30, with B symptoms	3 to 4 courses of ABVD + 30-Gy IFRT (grade A recommendation) OR 2 ABVD + 20-Gy IFRT in clinical trial setting (grade B recommendation)
American College of Radiology, 2008[23]	Stage I–II favorable disease: according to GHSG or EORTC criteria above	CMT (2–4 cycles of ABVD + 20-Gy to 30-Gy IFRT)

Abbreviations: EORTC, European Organisation for Research and Treatment of Cancer; GELA, Groupe d'Etude des Lymphomes de l'Adulte; GHSG, German Hodgkin Study Group; IFRT, involved-field radiation therapy; ISRT, involved site radiation therapy; M/T, mediastinum/thorax.

which were published in 2005 and described 5-year outcomes[24]; compared with the final reporting of that trial, these earlier results reported similar superiority of radiation-based therapy with respect to disease control with no differences in overall survival detected. Among guideline developers who do not recommend ABVD alone as a treatment option, reasons cited include the preliminary nature of the report describing 5-year outcomes, inferior disease-control outcomes associated with this therapy, the outdated nature of subtotal nodal RT received by patients in the HD.6 control arm, and the expectation that current use of IFRT is associated with a reduced risk of adverse late treatment effects.

COMPONENTS OF THE DECISION-MAKING PROCESS
Outcome Measures and Surrogates

Although overall survival coupled with health-related quality of life are likely the outcome measures of most importance to patients, clinical trials testing treatment strategies for populations with stage IA and IIA nonbulky Hodgkin lymphoma usually prioritize end points that measure disease control. The reasons for using these end points include the historical observation that disease control was a reasonable surrogate for overall survival and that earlier availability of robust disease-control data facilitated timely reporting. However, recent data show that progressive disease accounts for few deaths in patients with stage IA and IIA nonbulky Hodgkin lymphoma, even when median follow-ups are less than a decade (and thus do yet account for the additional late effects mortality that is observed in the second and third decades after treatment).[15–17] Therefore, although common, use of disease-control surrogate outcomes obtained with less than a decade of follow-up is associated with substantial risks if intended to be a proxy for long-term survival.

Compounding this generic limitation is the need for clarity around the problems associated with specific disease-control end points. For instance, a recommended end point is time to progression (TTP).[25] In calculating TTP, events contributing to this composite end point include the first of progressive Hodgkin lymphoma or death from Hodgkin lymphoma. The end point thus fails to capture deaths attributed to causes other than progressive Hodgkin lymphoma. Furthermore, given that stage IA and IIA nonbulky Hodgkin lymphoma is not associated with a sufficient disease burden to directly affect survival unless preceded by disease progression, all events associated with this end point are caused by disease progression.[26] Because most deaths in this population are unassociated with disease progression, TTP is not, nor can it be expected to be, an accurate surrogate for overall survival.

Another surrogate end point is progression-free survival (PFS), which is also a composite, in that events include the first of progressive Hodgkin lymphoma or death from any cause. This end point thus has the potential to account for deaths attributed to late treatment effects provided that the reporting of the clinical trial includes a duration of follow-up that is sufficient to span the period when late effects occur, and that the number (and thus relative proportion) of types of events (ie, progressive disease vs death from any cause) that comprise this composite are provided.[26–29] Without such clarity, PFS has also been shown to be an unreliable proxy for long-term overall survival.[16,17,26]

Practitioners and policy makers need to recognize the important differences that exist between debates around use of disease control end points as surrogates for overall survival in trials testing therapies for patients with metastatic carcinoma versus those evaluating patients with stage IA and IIA nonbulky Hodgkin lymphoma. In the former, any lack of surrogacy likely emphasizes the extreme precision of disease progression measurement associated with principles of conducting explanatory clinical trials,[30] especially within the context of limited survival durations; this limitation may be exaggerated when subsequent lines of therapy provide transient benefits. In contrast, for patients with stage IA to IIA nonbulky Hodgkin lymphoma, lack of surrogacy relates to deaths from causes other than progressive disease—an observation that is further compounded by knowledge that some of these deaths are related to the therapy received. Thus, the outcomes of interest that are associated with treatment policy determinations for these patients are associated with a unique paradigm that is distinct from considerations used for most other cancers: long-term overall survival is the outcome of greatest importance, data for this end point are largely unavailable for purported new therapeutic advances, and reliable proxy outcome measures that might facilitate estimates of the relative long-term survivals associated with competing options do not exist. Contributing to current dilemmas about outcome measures is the lack of published quality-of-life data from trials that compare approaches to management using CMT and ABVD alone. Evaluations of this end point, both during and after treatment, may assist in determining patient preferences.

Therapy that Includes Radiation

The background and rationale for choosing CMT that includes modern radiation treatment practices is detailed in the article by Marc André elsewhere in this issue. Recognizing that the options of CMT and ABVD alone are associated with relative risks and benefits, and trade-offs thus exist, we recognize several parameters that require consideration when choosing an overall treatment policy and implementing this policy in individual patients.

First, adverse late effects associated with wide-field radiation strategies, such as subtotal nodal and extended-field RT (EFRT), are well documented.[31] Examples include a population-based cancer registry study that includes 32,591 patients and identified significantly increased risks for all solid tumors; whereas chemotherapy alone resulted in an observed/expected ratio of 1.7, the ratio for patients receiving RT was 4.4 when follow-up was 20 to 24 years after diagnosis. Associations were observed between RT and risks for esophageal, gastric, rectal, female breast, bladder, thyroid, and bone/connective tissue malignancies.[32] That these risks exist with outdated RT strategies is well accepted and includes recognition that risks increase through at least the second and third decades of follow-up. The outcomes of patients in the HD.6 control arm, who received subtotal nodal RT, are consistent with these data. With a median follow-up of 4.2 years, there were 10 second cancers and 12 cardiac events in the 203 patients allocated to receive RT-containing therapy,[24] whereas with a median follow-up of 11.3 years, there were 23 and 26 events observed, respectively.[16]

Second, we recognize that when compared with outdated RT, modern RT includes reduced doses and smaller target volumes and is associated with reduced risks of late effects.[31] However, the magnitude of reduction remains uncertain and likely remains important. For instance, observations from the German Hodgkin Study Group (GHSG) HD8 trial, which randomly allocated patients to receive CMT that included EFRT or IFRT observed that with a median follow-up of 4.6 years, 24 of 532 (4.5%) patients assigned to EFRT and 15 of 532 (2.8%) assigned to IFRT had developed secondary malignancies[33]; with a median follow-up of 11 years, the incidence of second malignancies had increased to 58 (10.9%) and 45 (8.5%) events, respectively.[34] Although cardiac events were not tracked, the incidence of deaths attributed to cardiac causes showed a similar trend: at a median of 4.6 years, there were 5 and 7 cardiac deaths in the EFRT and IFRT groups, respectively, whereas with a median follow-up of 11 years, there were 15 and 12 such deaths. Thus, although risks are reduced with IFRT compared with EFRT, important risks of late effects seem to remain with IFRT, especially considering that the data on which this concern is based do not yet include follow-ups well into the second decade after treatment.

Third, we have previously reported our speculation that risks of late effects first become apparent in older patients.[19,26] This premise is based on the apparent increased risks of both death and nonfatal second cancers and cardiac events observed in patients allocated to receive RT in the HD.6 trial who were assigned to the unfavorable-risk cohort, a determination that included older age as a criterion,[16] and the observation that excess absolute risks of second cancers increase with attained age after treatment of Hodgkin lymphoma.[35] This premise is further suggested by outcomes observed in an individual patient cross-trial comparison of patients assigned to ABVD alone in HD.6 with patients assigned to the preferred arms of the GHSG HD10/11 trials; more deaths without previous progression of Hodgkin lymphoma were observed in older patients.[26] If true, our supposition means that patients younger than 40 years at diagnosis require follow-up well into the second, if not third, decade after therapy before risks of adverse late effects can be understood.

Excellent outcomes have been achieved with CMT strategies tested in the GHSG HD10 trial (8-year freedom from treatment failure of 86% with 2 cycles of ABVD and 20-Gy IFRT)[15] and the European Organization for Research and Treatment of Cancer (EORTC) H8 F trial (10-year event-free survival of 93% with 3 cycles of mechlorethamine, vincristine, procarbazine, and prednisone (MOPP) doxorubicin, bleomycin, vinblastine (ABV) and 36-Gy to 40-Gy IFRT).[11] These results establish a baseline for comparing new strategies that include involved nodal RT (INRT)[36] and involved site RT (ISRT)[37] radiation. However, although results from these 2 trials inform current recommendations, neither report includes median follow-up into the beginning of the second decade, let alone into the third decade after treatment, and median ages were 38.7 and 30 years, respectively, meaning that extended follow-up is needed to better understand the risks of late effects in younger patients. The relative merits of CMT strategies incorporating INRT and ISRT require similar scrutiny, with long-term follow-up of comparative data evaluating disease control and occurrence of late effects; given the time frames required, reports with such details are more than a decade away.

Therapy with Chemotherapy Alone

Systematic evaluations of a strategy to treat patients with stage IA and IIA nonbulky Hodgkin lymphoma with chemotherapy alone should consider only trials that test optimum chemotherapy (ie, ABVD). Thus, previous trials evaluating regimens such as MOPP (or its equivalents),[14] epirubicin, vinblastine, etoposide,[38] and epirubicin, bleomycin, vinblastine, and prednisone[39] do not provide data that contribute to current decision making. Similarly, a 2011 Cochrane review[40] does not assist policy determination, because this analysis included 3 such trials; the other 2 trials included did test ABVD but evaluated populations that included patients with stage III and bulky disease.

We have previously summarized the specifics and context of randomized trials comparing chemotherapy alone with strategies that include RT for patients with limited-stage Hodgkin lymphoma.[19,41] One of these reports described results of a MEDLINE search using PubMed from January 2002 to February 2007 and a review of abstracts from the American Society of Hematology (ASH) and American Society of Clinical Oncology (ASCO) annual meetings from 2002 to 2006. This search identified 3 randomized controlled trials (RCTs) testing ABVD alone in previously untreated adult patients with limited-stage Hodgkin lymphoma.[41] One of these trials was the initial report of HD.6,[24] one was a single institution comparison of ABVD with CMT in patients with stage I to IIA or B and stage IIIA disease,[42] and one was a subset analysis of a larger trial evaluating patients with all stages of Hodgkin lymphoma.[43] None of the trials detected differences in overall survival, and only the HD.6 trial had sufficient power to detect differences in disease control, which favored the group receiving RT. The premise that ABVD alone is associated with disease control that is approximately 7% worse than CMT approaches comes from these data.

We repeated this PubMed search in May 2013 using the MESH term Hodgkin and the limiting terms "randomized controlled trials" and "meta-analysis" to identify publications since February 2007; 231 citations were identified and reviewed. After excluding articles that were not phase III RCTs or meta-analyses testing ABVD-based chemotherapy alone as initial therapy for patients with nonbulky stage IA and IIA Hodgkin lymphoma, 3 publications remained. These publications included the final analysis of HD.6 described earlier,[16] the Cochrane meta-analysis referred to above,[40] and a pediatric study testing cyclophosphamide, vincristine, prednisone, and procarbazine/ABV therapy alone.[44] Furthermore, we reviewed ASH abstracts from 2007 to 2012 and identified 2 additional RCTs: the UK National Cancer Research Institute RAPID (PET Scan in Planning Treatment in Patients Undergoing Combination Chemotherapy For Stage IA or Stage IIA Hodgkin Lymphoma)[17] and EORTC-led H10[18] trials, which both tested response-adapted strategies using positron emission tomography (PET).

We have previously provided our interpretation of the important conclusions associated with HD.6 data.[19] First, superior 12-year overall survival (94% vs 87%) was observed with ABVD alone, and this difference was caused by more deaths in the RT arm from causes other than progressive Hodgkin lymphoma or early treatment complication; it is recognized that these results are contributed to by use of an outdated RT strategy. Second, the 12-year outcomes of patients assigned to ABVD alone, overall survival of 94%, and freedom from disease progression of 87%, are considered to be excellent and comparable with those reported in randomized trials testing CMT that includes IFRT. Third, the observation that the risk of disease progression with chemotherapy alone was almost twice that associated with treatment that includes RT (HR = 1.91), whereas the risk of death was reduced by half (HR = 0.5), refutes use of disease-control measures as an accurate proxy for overall survival in this patient population. Among patients in the ABVD-alone cohort who were evaluable for response after 2 treatment cycles (90% of patients), those with a complete remission (CR) or unconfirmed complete remission (CRu) had superior 12-year disease control (94% vs 81%; HR = 0.28; P = .02) and a trend to superior 12-year overall survival (98% vs 92%; HR = 0.17; P = .06) when compared with those not achieving a CR/CRu status; these data provide a basis of support to test response-adapted therapy using PET.

The UK RAPID and EORTC-led H10 trials have been reported in preliminary abstract form and provide insights about PET-directed response-adapted therapy and comparisons of chemotherapy alone with CMT. Using a noninferiority design, the RAPID trial enrolled 602 patients with stage IA and IIA nonbulky Hodgkin lymphoma between 2003 and 2010.[17] All patients received 3 cycles of ABVD followed by centrally reviewed PET. Those with a scan deemed to be consistent with potential persisting disease received a fourth cycle of ABVD and IFRT. Those with a negative scan were randomized to receive IFRT and no further treatment. Of the 426 patients with a negative scan (75% of those accrued), 420 were randomized and included in an intent-to-treat analysis that reported 3-year PFS of 90.7% among those receiving ABVD alone and 93.8% among those randomized to receive IFRT. This difference of –2.9% was associated with 95% CIs of –10.7% and +1.4% and thus exceeded the prespecified noninferiority boundary of –7%. The 3-year overall survivals were 99.5% among those allocated to ABVD alone and 97% among those allocated to IFRT. The investigators concluded that patients with a negative PET scan after 3 cycles of ABVD do not require IFRT, chemotherapy alone reduces treatment time and costs, improves tolerability, and removes the burden of early and late radiation-associated toxicities.[17] Given the noninferiority design, subsequent reporting also include the results of a per-protocol analysis.

The H10[18] trial began accruing patients ages 15 to 70 years with newly diagnosed supradiaphragmatic stage I to II classic Hodgkin lymphoma in 2006; our synopsis is confined to the favorable-risk population who were identified as having fewer than 4 nodal areas of disease with no areas of bulky disease, ages younger than 50 years, and ESR less than 30 with B symptoms or less than 50 without B symptoms (the H10F trial). All patients underwent PET after 2 cycles of ABVD; patients randomized to a control arm received 3 cycles of ABVD and 30-Gy INRT without consideration of PET results, whereas those in the experimental arm received PET-directed therapy. Patients in the experimental arm with negative PET scan received 2 additional cycles of ABVD (total of 4 cycles) and those with a positive scan received 2 cycles of escalated-dose BEACOPP and 30-Gy INRT. Of 444 patients, 381 (86%) were deemed to be PET negative; the 1-year PFS outcomes were 94.9% with ABVD alone and 100% with CMT (HR 9.36, 95% CI 2.45, 35.73). These findings led an independent Data Safety Monitoring Committee to recommend that the trial be halted, including with an explanation that the a priori null hypothesis for noninferiority would not be rejected.

Although determination of practice policies requires results from properly designed and executed RCTs, nonrandomized comparisons may contribute additional context and allow for hypothesis generation. The NCIC CTG and GHSG have thus conducted an individual patient cross-trial comparison[26] evaluating 588 patients who would have been mutually eligible for the HD.6 trial and either the GHSG HD10[15] or HD11 trial[45] (Fig. 1, Table 2).[26] The 8-year TTP was superior and PFS trended toward superiority in the GHSG cohort, who were assigned to CMT. No differences in 8-year overall survival were apparent (95% in both cohorts). With a median follow-up of 11.2 years, 10 deaths were observed in 182 patients in the HD.6 cohort, 5 from Hodgkin lymphoma or immediate treatment toxicity and 5 from other causes; with a median follow-up of 7.6 years, 19 deaths were observed in 406 patients in the GHSG cohort, 7 from Hodgkin lymphoma or immediate treatment toxicity and 12 from other causes. All TTP events were caused by disease progression. Of the 27 PFS events in HD.6, 23 were caused by disease progression and 4 were deaths without previous disease progression; of the 38 PFS events in the GHSG cohorts, 25 were caused by disease progression and 13 were deaths without previous disease progression. A subset analysis of those eligible for HD10 suggested that disease-control benefits associated with CMT may be limited to those not achieving CR/CRu, as assessed by physical examination and computed tomographic scanning. Among those assessed as achieving a CR/CRu after 2 cycles of ABVD, the respective 8-year TTP and overall survivals were 95% and 100% in the HD.6 cohort and 93% and 96% in the HD10 cohort. In contrast, among those assessed as not achieving a CR/CRu after 2 cycles of ABVD, the respective 8-year TTP and overall survivals were 78% and 91% in the HD.6 cohort and 92% and 95% in the HD10 cohort.

In Table 3, the relevant parameters associated with these comparative reports evaluating response-adapted therapy are summarized. Important differences include the randomized and nonrandomized designs, the median durations of follow-up, the patient populations included, the timing of response assessment, the modality for assessing response, and the determinants for a positive or negative result. These

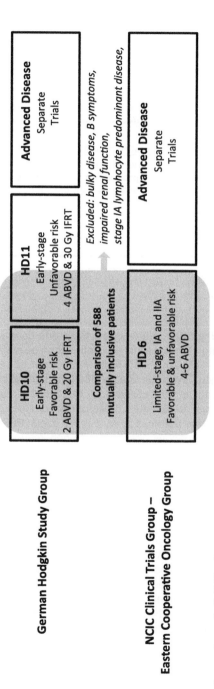

German Hodgkin Study Group

HD10
Early-stage
Favorable risk
2 ABVD & 20 Gy IFRT

HD11
Early-stage
Unfavorable risk
4 ABVD & 30 Gy IFRT

Advanced Disease
Separate
Trials

**Comparison of 588
mutually inclusive patients**

*Excluded: bulky disease, B symptoms,
impaired renal function,
stage IA lymphocyte predominant disease,*

**NCIC Clinical Trials Group –
Eastern Cooperative Oncology Group**

HD.6
Limited-stage, IA and IIA
Favorable & unfavorable risk
4-6 ABVD

Advanced Disease
Separate
Trials

Fig. 1. Comparison of eligibility for GHSG HD10 and HD11 and NCIC CTG-ECOG HD.6 clinical trials.[26]

Table 2
Cross-trial comparison showing events contributing to clinical trial end points at 8 years of follow-up, in 588 patients with stage IA to IIA favorable-risk Hodgkin lymphoma

GHSG HD10/11 ABVD + IFRT N = 406	NCIC CTG-ECOG HD.6 ABVD Alone N = 182	HR (95% CI)
TTP		
Composite end point at which event is first of progression or death from Hodgkin lymphoma		
93%, all 25 events were disease progression	87%, all 23 events were disease progression	0.44 (0.24, 0.78)
PFS		
Composite end point at which event is first of progression or death from any cause		
89%, 25 events were disease progression, 13 events were death without previous progression	86%, 23 events were disease progression, 4 events were death without previous progression	0.71 (0.42, 1.18)
Overall survival Event is death from any cause		
95%, 19 events	95%, 10 events	1.09 (0.49, 2.40)

Data from Hay AE, Klimm B, Chen BE, et al. An individual patient-data comparison of combined-modality therapy and ABVD alone for patients with limited-stage Hodgkin lymphoma. Ann Oncol 2013. [Epub ahead of print].

variations likely explain the major differences in the proportions of patients deemed to have achieved a CR state at the specific evaluation time point, with values of 40% in the HD.6 trial, 62% in the HD10 trial, 75% in the RAPID trial, and 86% in the H10F trial. Across these reports, there are considerable differences of the benchmark time point used for end point comparison (PFS assessed at 1, 3, and 8 years) and the durations of median follow-up. However, allowing for these differences, use of response-adapted strategies seems to have the potential to narrow the gap in PFS differences between ABVD alone and CMT approaches observed with non–response-adapted strategies from 7% to less than 5%. Based on these data and previous results observed with evaluations of non–response-adapted strategies, it seems highly unlikely that overall survival will be inferior with ABVD alone used according to a response-adapted strategy; given uncertainties associated with the frequency of late effects that may be observed during the second and third decades of follow-up of patients treated with CMT that incorporates modern RT strategies, the potential for superior overall survival using a strategy of ABVD alone is plausible. Necessary parameters for long-term overall survival to be superior with ABVD alone include accounting for late effects associated with an increased use of second-line therapy, which is likely to be required in up to 5% of patients, and assurances that with long-term follow-up, more frequent late disease recurrence is not observed.

These data do not include patients with bulky disease. Furthermore, these data either directly support, or are consistent with, a recommendation that patients who do not enter a CR/CRu status with midtreatment evaluation should receive RT.

THE PRESENT AND FUTURE

Based on the data discussed in this article, we recommend that new patients with stage IA and IIA nonbulky Hodgkin lymphoma be presented with the option to receive

Table 3
Outcomes of comparative reports testing response-adapted strategies in patients with stage IA to IIA nonbulky Hodgkin lymphoma

	Type of Study	Response Assessment	CR Rate (%)	Point Estimate (y)	PFS of Patients Achieving Early CR (%)		Overall Survival of Patients Achieving Early CR (%)	
					ABVD Alone	CMT	ABVD Alone	CMT
RAPID (UK)	RCT	Negative PET after 3 ABVD	75	3	90.7	93.8	99.5	97
EORTC-led H10F	RCT	Negative PET after 2 ABVD	86	1	94.9	100	100	100
NCIC CTG-ECOG HD.6 and GHSG HD10	Nonrandomized cohort comparison	Negative CT after 2 ABVD	40 (HD.6) 62 (HD10)	8	95	93	100	96

Abbreviations: CT, computed tomography; CR, complete remission.

treatment with a strategy that has as its intent therapy with ABVD alone. The advantages of this strategy include high expectations of disease control, avoidance of radiation-related late effects, and, based on high-quality data, expectations of at least comparable overall survival. This strategy should be implemented according to a response-adapted paradigm with midtreatment evaluation of disease response using PET. We recognize that this strategy is shaped by the HD.6 trial, which evaluated outdated RT technology, the preliminary nature of the data associated with the RAPID and H10F trials and the nonrandomized design of the HD.6 to HD10/11 comparison. We also recognize that there are remaining uncertainties about the optimum timing of midtreatment evaluation (eg, after 2 vs after 3 treatment cycles) and the specifics associated with determining PET positivity versus negativity. Long-term disease control with initial therapy according to this strategy may be inferior to a CMT strategy, but we expect the margin of inferiority to be less than 5% and that this risk will be compensated by avoidance of late effects that are attributed to RT. In discussing this option with patients, careful presentation of a CMT option is also required, and these options are best presented through multidisciplinary collaborations, which include a hematologist or medical oncologist and a radiation oncologist.

We expect that future advances will include refinements in identifying patient populations through use of predictive biomarkers,[46] with potential candidates including three-dimensional telomere signatures,[47] macrophagelike genetic signatures of Hodgkin Reed-Sternberg cells[48] and plasma Epstein-Barr virus DNA levels.[49] Refinements in response assessment will also include these laboratory-based biomarkers and applications of new imaging technologies (eg, new PET ligands) that include understandings of optimum timing and standardization of response assessment. We expect that RT technologies will continue to evolve so that disease control can be maximized and treatment of normal structures is minimized[50,51] and that new systemic therapies that include targeted agents, such as brentuximab,[52] will provide new options to current therapies. These future opportunities will require high-quality clinical trials and multidisciplinary collaboration and must account for a fundamental paradigm associated with this patient population, which is the importance of long-term outcomes and our limitations in appreciating all details of how these are affected by treatment choices.

REFERENCES

1. Gall EA. The surgical treatment of malignant lymphoma. Ann Surg 1943;118(6): 1064–70.
2. Pack GT, Molander DW. The surgical treatment of Hodgkin's disease. Cancer Res 1966;26(6 Part 1):1254–63.
3. Gilbert R, Babaianta L. Notre methode de roentgentherapie da la lymphogranulomatose (Hodgkin): resultats eloignes. Acta Radiol 1931;12(6):523–9 [in French].
4. Peters MV. A study of survivals in Hodgkin's disease treated radiologically. Am J Roentgenol Radium Ther 1950;63:299–311.
5. Kaplan HS. The radical radiotherapy of regionally localized Hodgkin's disease. Radiology 1962;78:553–61.
6. Carde P, Burgers JM, Henry-Amar M, et al. Clinical stages I and II Hodgkin's disease: a specifically tailored therapy according to prognostic factors. J Clin Oncol 1988;6(2):239–52.
7. Tubiana M, Henry-Amar M, Hayat M, et al. The EORTC treatment of early stages of Hodgkin's disease: the role of radiotherapy. Int J Radiat Oncol Biol Phys 1984; 10(2):197–210.

8. Dameshek W, Weisfuse L, Stein T. Nitrogen mustard in Hodgkin's disease: analysis of fifty consecutive cases. Blood 1949;4(4):338–79.
9. Devita JR, Serpick AA, Carbone PP. Combination chemotherapy in the treatment of advanced Hodgkin's disease. Ann Intern Med 1970;73(6):881–95.
10. Engert A, Franklin J, Eich HT, et al. Two cycles of doxorubicin, bleomycin, vinblastine, and dacarbazine plus extended-field radiotherapy is superior to radiotherapy alone in early favorable Hodgkin's lymphoma: final results of the GHSG HD7 Trial. J Clin Oncol 2007;25(23):3495–502.
11. Ferme C, Eghbali H, Meerwaldt JH, et al. Chemotherapy plus involved-field radiation in early-stage Hodgkin's disease. N Engl J Med 2007;357(19):1916–27.
12. Press OW, LeBlanc M, Lichter AS, et al. Phase III randomized Intergroup trial of subtotal lymphoid irradiation versus doxorubicin, vinblastine, and subtotal lymphoid irradiation for stage IA to IIA Hodgkin's disease. J Clin Oncol 2001; 19(22):4238–44.
13. Henry-Amar M, Aeppli DM, Anderson J. Long term survival and study of causes of death. In: Somers R, Henry-Amar M, Meerwaldt JK, Carde P, editors. Treatment strategy in Hodgkin's disease. London: John Libbey; 1990. p. 381–418.
14. Carde P, Hagenbeek A, Hayat M, et al. Clinical staging versus laparotomy and combined modality with MOPP versus ABVD in early-stage Hodgkin's disease: the H6 twin randomized trials from the European Organization for Research and Treatment of Cancer Lymphoma Cooperative Group. J Clin Oncol 1993;11(11):2258–72.
15. Engert A, Plutschow A, Eich HT, et al. Reduced treatment intensity in patients with early-stage Hodgkin's lymphoma. N Engl J Med 2010;363(7):640–52.
16. Meyer RM, Gospodarowicz MK, Connors JM, et al. ABVD alone versus radiation-based therapy in limited-stage Hodgkin's lymphoma. N Engl J Med 2011;366(5):399–408.
17. Radford J, Barrington S, Counsell N, et al. Involved field radiotherapy versus no further treatment in patients with clinical stages IA and IIA Hodgkin lymphoma and a 'negative' PET scan after 3 cycles ABVD. Results of the UK NCRI RAPID Trial. ASH Annual Meeting Abstracts 2012;120(21):547.
18. Andre MP, Reman O, Federico M, et al. Interim analysis of the randomized EORTC/LYSA/FIL Intergroup H10 trial on early PET-scan driven treatment adaptation in stage I/II Hodgkin lymphoma. ASH Annual Meeting Abstracts 2012; 120(21):549.
19. Meyer RM, Hoppe RT. Point/counterpoint: early-stage Hodgkin lymphoma and the role of radiation therapy. Blood 2012;120(23):4488–95.
20. NCCN clinical practice guidelines in oncology: Hodgkin lymphoma. National Comprehensive Cancer Network. 2013;(Version 2). Available at: http://www.nccn.org/. Accessed September 8, 2013.
21. Eichenauer DA, Engert A, Dreyling M, On behalf of the ESMO Guidelines Working Group. Hodgkin's lymphoma: ESMO Clinical Practice Guidelines for diagnosis, treatment and follow-up. Ann Oncol 2011;22(Suppl 6):vi55–8.
22. Brusamolino E, Bacigalupo A, Barosi G, et al. Classical Hodgkin's lymphoma in adults: guidelines of the Italian Society of Hematology, the Italian Society of Experimental Hematology, and the Italian Group for Bone Marrow Transplantation on initial work-up, management, and follow-up. Haematologica 2009; 94(4):550–65.
23. Das P, Ng A, Constine LS, et al. ACR Appropriateness criteria; Hodgkin's lymphoma–favorable prognosis stage I and II. American College of Radiology, 2008; Available at: http://www.guideline.gov/content.aspx?id=32633&search=hodgkin+lymphoma. Accessed September 8, 2013.

24. Meyer RM, Gospodarowicz MK, Connors JM, et al. Randomized comparison of ABVD chemotherapy with a strategy that includes radiation therapy in patients with limited-stage Hodgkin's lymphoma: National Cancer Institute of Canada Clinical Trials Group and the Eastern Cooperative Oncology Group. J Clin Oncol 2005;23(21):4634–42.

25. Cheson BD, Pfistner B, Juweid ME, et al. Revised response criteria for malignant lymphoma. J Clin Oncol 2007;25(5):579–86.

26. Hay AE, Klimm B, Chen BE, et al. An individual patient-data comparison of combined-modality therapy and ABVD alone for patients with limited-stage Hodgkin lymphoma. Ann Oncol 2013. [Epub ahead of print].

27. Wu L, Cook RJ. Misspecification of Cox regression models with composite endpoints. Stat Med 2012;31(28):3545–62.

28. Pfirrmann M, Hochhaus A, Lauseker M, et al. Recommendations to meet statistical challenges arising from endpoints beyond overall survival in clinical trials on chronic myeloid leukemia. Leukemia 2011;25(9):1433–8.

29. Freemantle N, Calvert M, Wood J, et al. Composite outcomes in randomized trials: greater precision but with greater uncertainty? JAMA 2003;289(19):2554–9.

30. Meyer RM. Contrasting explanatory and pragmatic randomized controlled trials in oncology. American Society Clinical Oncology Annual Meeting Book. Chicago, June 3-7, 2011. p. 31.

31. Hodgson DC. Late effects in the era of modern therapy for Hodgkin lymphoma. Hematology Am Soc Hematol Educ Program 2011;2011(1):323–9.

32. Dores GM, Metayer C, Curtis RE, et al. Second malignant neoplasms among long-term survivors of Hodgkin's disease: a population-based evaluation over 25 years. J Clin Oncol 2002;20(16):3484–94.

33. Engert A, Schiller P, Josting A, et al. Involved-field radiotherapy is equally effective and less toxic compared with extended-field radiotherapy after four cycles of chemotherapy in patients with early-stage unfavorable Hodgkin's lymphoma: results of the HD8 Trial of the German Hodgkin's Lymphoma Study Group. J Clin Oncol 2003;21(19):3601–8.

34. Sasse S, Klimm B, Goergen H, et al. Comparing long-term toxicity and efficacy of combined modality treatment including extended- or involved-field radiotherapy in early-stage Hodgkin's lymphoma. Ann Oncol 2012;23(11):2953–9.

35. Hodgson DC, Gilbert ES, Dores GM, et al. Long-term solid cancer risk among 5-year survivors of Hodgkin's lymphoma. J Clin Oncol 2007;25(12):1489–97.

36. Campbell BA, Voss N, Pickles T, et al. Involved-nodal radiation therapy as a component of combination therapy for limited-stage Hodgkin's lymphoma: a question of field size. J Clin Oncol 2008;26(32):5170–4.

37. Specht L, Yahalom J, Illidge T, et al. Modern radiation therapy for Hodgkin lymphoma: field and dose guidelines from the International Lymphoma Radiation Oncology Group (ILROG). Int J Radiat Oncol Biol Phys, in press.

38. Pavone V, Ricardi U, Luminari S, et al. ABVD plus radiotherapy versus EVE plus radiotherapy in unfavorable stage IA and IIA Hodgkin's lymphoma: results from an Intergruppo Italiano Linfomi randomized study. Ann Oncol 2008;19(4):763–8.

39. Noordijk EM, Carde P, Dupouy N, et al. Combined-modality therapy for clinical stage I or II Hodgkin's lymphoma: long-term results of the European Organisation for Research and Treatment of Cancer H7 Randomized Controlled Trials. J Clin Oncol 2006;24(19):3128–35.

40. Herbst C, Rehan F, Skoetz N, et al. Chemotherapy alone versus chemotherapy plus radiotherapy for early stage Hodgkin lymphoma. Cochrane Database Syst Rev 2011;(2):CD007110.

41. Meyer RM. Selected management issues of patients with Hodgkin lymphoma. In: Crowther MA, Ginsberg J, Schunemann HJ, et al, editors. Evidence-based hematology. 1st edition. Chichester, West Sussex, UK: Wiley-Blackwell; 2008. p. 365–71.
42. Straus DJ, Portlock CS, Qin J, et al. Results of a prospective randomized clinical trial of doxorubicin, bleomycin, vinblastine, and dacarbazine (ABVD) followed by radiation therapy (RT) versus ABVD alone for stages I, II, and IIIA nonbulky Hodgkin disease. Blood 2004;104(12):3483–9.
43. Laskar S, Gupta T, Vimal S, et al. Consolidation radiation after complete remission in Hodgkin's disease following six cycles of doxorubicin, bleomycin, vinblastine, and dacarbazine chemotherapy: is there a need? J Clin Oncol 2004;22(1):62–8.
44. Wolden SL, Chen L, Kelly KM, et al. Long-term results of CCG 5942: a randomized comparison of chemotherapy with and without radiotherapy for children with Hodgkin's lymphoma: a report from the Children's Oncology Group. J Clin Oncol 2012;30(26):3174–80.
45. Eich HT, Diehl V, Goergen H, et al. Intensified chemotherapy and dose-reduced involved-field radiotherapy in patients with early unfavorable Hodgkin's lymphoma: final analysis of the German Hodgkin Study Group HD11 Trial. J Clin Oncol 2010;28(27):4199–206.
46. Meyer RM. EBV DNA: a Hodgkin lymphoma biomarker? Blood 2013;121(18):3541–2.
47. Knecht H, Kongruttanachok N, Sawan B, et al. Three-dimensional telomere signatures of Hodgkin- and Reed-Sternberg cells at diagnosis identify patients with poor response to conventional chemotherapy. Transl Oncol 2012;5(4):269–77.
48. Steidl C, Diepstra A, Lee T, et al. Gene expression profiling of microdissected Hodgkin Reed-Sternberg cells correlates with treatment outcome in classical Hodgkin lymphoma. Blood 2012;120(17):3530–40.
49. Kanakry JA, Li H, Gellert LL, et al. Plasma Epstein-Barr virus DNA predicts outcome in advanced Hodgkin lymphoma: correlative analysis from a large North American co-operative group trial. Blood 2013;121(18):3547–53.
50. Hoppe BS, Flampouri S, Su Z, et al. Effective Dose reduction to cardiac structures using protons compared with 3DCRT and IMRT in mediastinal Hodgkin lymphoma. Int J Radiat Oncol Biol Phys 2012;84(2):449–55.
51. Fiandra CF, Filippi AR, Catuzzo P, et al. Different IMRT solutions vs. 3D-conformal radiotherapy in early stage Hodgkin's lymphoma: dosimetric comparison and clinical considerations. Radiat Oncol 2012;7:186.
52. Younes A, Gopal AK, Smith SE, et al. Results of a pivotal phase II study of brentuximab vedotin for patients with relapsed or refractory Hodgkin's lymphoma. J Clin Oncol 2012;30(18):2183–9.

Early Intensification Treatment Approach in Advanced-stage Hodgkin Lymphoma

Peter Borchmann, MD, PhD

KEYWORDS

- Hodgkin lymphoma • BEACOPP • Overall survival • Evidence

KEY POINTS

- No significant or only relevant differences have been documented in randomized trials between ABVD and BEACOPP$_{escalated}$ with regard to acute treatment-related mortality, second solid tumors, second acute myeloid leukemia, or any other late toxicities. However, data from non-controlled studies suggest a more pronounced gonadal toxicity with BEACOPP$_{escalated}$.
- The patient's perspective on the importance of gonadal toxicity as compared with the importance of being cured must not be ignored. Also, the patient's perspective regarding the importance of not experiencing relapse from their malignant disease must not be ignored.
- Regarding antilymphoma efficacy, the 5-year progression-free survival for advanced-stage Hodgkin lymphoma patients up to 60 years old treated with BEACOPP$_{escalated}$ is approximately 90%. This is about 20% better than the results with ABVD.
- With 6 cycles of BEACOPP$_{escalated}$ as first-line treatment, overall survival at 5 years is 95%. This is 10% better than ABVD as initial treatment as confirmed in a meta-analysis providing highest level of evidence.
- Both physicians and patients must be aware of the meaningfully higher risk of death at 5 years already when using ABVD as first-line treatment. Whenever the health care setting allows administering BEACOPP$_{escalated}$, the progressionfree and overall survival benefit clearly advocate this intensified first-line treatment as standard of care.

INTRODUCTION

Hodgkin lymphoma (HL) is among the most common malignancies in young adults. Survival has substantially increased over the last decades, even for patients in the advanced stages. How to balance risks and benefits of different treatment strategies, however, still remains a matter of controversy. The key question is, should intensified chemotherapy be applied upfront or should it be reserved for relapsing patients.[1] The early intensification approach aims at curing as many patients as possible with

Disclosures: None.
1st Department of Internal Medicine, German Hodgkin Study Group, University Hospital Cologne, Kerpener Straße 62, 50924 Koeln, Germany
E-mail address: peter.borchmann@uni-koeln.de

Hematol Oncol Clin N Am 28 (2014) 65–74
http://dx.doi.org/10.1016/j.hoc.2013.10.002
0889-8588/14/$ – see front matter © 2014 Elsevier Inc. All rights reserved.

an aggressive first-line chemotherapy.[2] This approach is standard of care in European HL study groups such as the German Hodgkin Study Group (GHSG), The Lymphoma Study Association, and the European Organisation for Research and Treatment of Cancer. Standard regimen is 6 cycles of BEACOPP$_{escalated}$ (bleomycin, etoposide, doxorubicin, cyclophosphamide, vincristine, procarbazine, prednisone) followed by radiotherapy to metabolic active residual disease. This approach induces high progression-free and overall survival rates (PFS, OS), but exposes patients to considerable acute chemotherapy-related toxicity.[2] Because the discussion on its efficacy and toxicity profile as compared with initial treatment with ABVD (doxorubicin, bleomycin, vinblastine, dacarbazine) has been and still is emotional and sometimes reflects more individual beliefs than currently available knowledge,[3–5] this article aims at summarizing the most important facts on BEACOPP$_{escalated}$ derived from randomized trials.

EFFICACY: PFS AND OS
HD9

BEACOPP$_{escalated}$ reflects the introduction of granulocyte-colonystimulating factor (G-CSF) in hematology. In the 1980s it was hypothesized that dose density might increase the response rate of chemotherapy-sensitive tumors. Dirk Hasenclever developed a statistical model of the association of tumor growth kinetics and the effects of chemotherapy. The model was used to simulate the effect of dose escalation, dose density, and schedule changes in the COPP/ABVD regimen. This simulation demonstrated that the most potent effect would be achieved through dose escalation of cytostatics. This effect was estimated at an increase of 10% to 15% in PFS after 5 years. From this model, the BEACOPP regimen with G-CSF support was developed and tested versus the former standard COPP/ABVD in the HD9 study.[2] The HD9 study randomized 1195 patients in 3 treatment groups (COPP/ABVD, BEACOPP$_{baseline}$, and BEACOPP$_{escalated}$) and clearly demonstrated the superiority of BEACOPP$_{escalated}$. The 10-year data for this study have confirmed the initial results: the freedom from treatment failure and OS rates for COPP/ABVD were 74% and 75%, respectively, after 120 months. The corresponding results for BEACOPP$_{escalated}$ are 82% and 86%, respectively.[6] OS is thus 11% better than with standard COPP/ABVD. This effect is particularly pronounced in the group of patients with an intermediate risk profile according to the international prognostic score (IPS 2-3), which also forms the largest subgroup of patients (IPS 0-1: 28%, IPS 2-3: 38%, IPS 4-7: 13%).

HD12

However, the toxicity of 8 cycles of BEACOPP$_{escalated}$ is high. In addition to the considerable acute toxicity, the development of secondary acute leukemia prompted concern. In the HD9 study, the incidence of secondary acute leukemia was 3% compared with only 0.4% in the COPP/ABVD arm. The follow-up study HD12 therefore looked at reducing the chemotherapy to 4 cycles of BEACOPP$_{escalated}$ followed by 4 cycles of BEACOPP$_{baseline}$ ("4+4" regimen).[7] At 5 years, there were no significant differences regarding OS or PFS, although there was a decrease in absolute numbers with the 4+4 regimen. Importantly, the incidence of severe toxicities could not be reduced by the reduction of chemotherapy, so 8 cycles of BEACOPP$_{escalated}$ remained standard of care in the GHSG.

HD15

In the subsequent study, de-escalation of chemotherapy was investigated with a reduction in the number of escalated cycles from 8 to 6 and with the introduction of a dose dense BEACOPP$_{baseline}$ regimen (BEACOPP-14).[8] The study was designed to show noninferiority of the experimental treatment groups. In addition, positron emission tomography (PET)-guided radiotherapy of residual disease ≥2.5 cm was investigated. Only PET-positive patients received consolidating radiotherapy. A total of 2182 patients were randomized among the 3 study arms. Surprisingly, when comparing 6 cycles of BEACOPP$_{escalated}$ with 8 cycles, both PFS (90.3% vs 85.6%) and OS (95.3% vs 91.9%) were significantly superior with the reduced number of cycles. With regard to radiotherapy, the negative predictive value for PET at 12 months was 94.1% (95% CI 92.1%–96.1%) and only 11% of all patients received additional radiotherapy without compromising the tumor control.[9] It is thus safe not to irradiate patients with residual tumor masses ≥2.5 cm, if they are PET negative. In summary, the HD15 established 6 cycles of BEACOPP$_{escalated}$ as a new standard of care based on a significantly improved PFS and OS.[10]

HD18

The idea of this trial is to reduce the number of chemotherapy cycles further from 6 to 4 in patients with a PET-negative response after 2 cycles of BEACOPP$_{escalated}$ (early interim PET). If this reduction could be done without a loss of efficacy, it would be a major improvement for the patients. The cumulative dose of alkylating agents after 4 cycles of BEACOPP$_{escalated}$ should be low enough to improve the toxicity profile of the early intensification approach significantly. The study is still enrolling patients and results for this part of the study will not be available before 2018. Another question to be answered by this study is related to patients with PET-positive disease at early interim staging. These patients have received additional treatment with the anti-CD20 antibody rituximab to improve their outcome. Results for this part of the HD18 trial will be available at the end of 2013. It might be noted though that the response adapted de-escalation of therapy using an early interim PET has never been shown to be safe in a randomized trial so far. Thus, without evidence from randomized trials, early interim PET must currently not be used to guide therapy outside clinical studies in advanced-stage disease.

ACUTE AND LONG-TERM TOXICITIES

Acute Toxicity

Thousands of patients have been treated with BEACOPP$_{escalated}$ within controlled international multicenter trials. This review refers to the experience derived from the GHSG studies. These trials include large tertiary cancer centers, but more than half of the patients within the GHSG trials are enrolled by small centers and private practitioners enrolling about one patient per year. In this real-life setting, 94% of all patients experience at least one World Health Organization toxicity grade III/IV.

Leukopenia

Leukopenia is observed in almost 90% of patients; anemia and thrombocytopenia are observed in about 50% of patients.[2,7,8] Consequently, infections are documented in around 20% to 25% of patients. Acute treatment-related mortality (TRM) of 6 cycles of BEACOPP$_{escalated}$ varied from 0.8% up to 2.5%.[8] TRM highly depends on 2 easily assessable patient-related risk factors: age and performance status. Patients ≤40 years old show a TRM of only 0.7%; however, this risk increases to 2.5% in patients between 40 and 49 years, 3.8% in those between 50 and 59, and 14.3% in patients aged older than 60 years.[11] Furthermore, a poor performance status increases the risk of TRM. Thus, the TRM risk can be evaluated easily and patients at risk can be monitored adequately. In the ongoing HD18 study prophylactic measures have been implemented including obligatory antibiotic treatment during neutropenia and TRM is less than 1% with more than 1000 patients enrolled so far.

Organ toxicity is observed in almost all organ systems but with very low frequencies. An exception to this rule is severe peripheral neuropathy due to the use of vincristine, occurring in up to 10% of patients.

Gonadal Toxicity

Gonadal toxicity must be mentioned. Karolin Behringer has investigated this important question in the G5 (ie, GHSG studies HD13, HD14, and HD15).[12] A total of 1323 (55%) of 2412 contacted female and male survivors were evaluable for analysis (mean follow-up 46 and 48 months, respectively). After 6 to 8 cycles of BEACOPP, menstrual activity was strongly related to age (<30 years: 82% vs >30 years: 45%; $P<.001$; prolonged recovery time up to 3 years). Thirty-four percent of women older than 30 years suffered severe menopausal symptoms (3- to 4-fold more frequently than expected). In contrast, male survivors had mean levels of testosterone within the normal range and reported no increased symptoms of hypogonadism. However, in men follicle-stimulating hormone and inhibin-B levels indicated infertility for most survivors regardless of age. Importantly, for both men and women, the sexual quality of life was shown to be more closely related to patient characteristics and sexual functions before start of treatment than to the intensity of treatment. Sexual functions recover in most patients after the end of treatment.[13]

Thus, there is well-grounded information on gonadal toxicity of BEACOPP$_{escalated}$ regarding sexual functions, hypogonadism, and infertility. It is important to note that all of these side effects depend on age and gender. Therefore, the individual who wishes to avoid gonadal damage can be balanced against the individual who wishes to be cured with the primary treatment and not to experience the psychological stress of relapsing from the lymphoma and being in need of a very demanding second-line treatment. Publications suggest that physicians might overestimate the meaning of infertility for patients suffering from HL and, accordingly, underestimate the meaning of relapse-free survival for these patients.[1,14]

Long-Term Toxicity

Little is known about the long-term toxicities of BEACOPP$_{escalated}$. Second malignancies including non-HL, solid tumors, and acute myeloid leukemia (sAML/myelodysplastic syndrome [MDS]) were the focus when BEACOPP was introduced. At 5-year median follow-up, there were 0.4% cases of sAML/MDS in the COPP/ABVD group, 0.8% in the BEACOPP baseline group, and 1.9% in the BEACOPP escalated group.[2] At 10-years median follow-up, there were 0.4%, 1.5%, and 3.0% of patients with sAML/MDS.[6] The total number of second malignancies was not different between the 3 treatment arms. Interestingly, the risk of sAML/MDS after BEACOPP escalated was only 0.9% at 4 years in the HD12 study.[7] It is known that radiotherapy combined with chemotherapy add to the risk for second malignancies. In HD9, 70% of patients received additional radiation, whereas in HD12, only 38% of 1502 patients enrolled were irradiated. The reduction of radiotherapy very likely contributes to an improved safety profile in HL patients, which is certainly also true for the cumulative dose of the alkylating agents cyclophosphamide and procarbazine. With 6 cycles of BEACOP-P$_{escalated}$ instead of 8 cycles in the GHSG HD15 trial (and only 11% of patients receiving consolidating radiotherapy), the risk of sAML/MDS decreased to 0.3%.[8] So far, no increased risk for solid tumors has been detected. The median observation time of 10 years for BEACOPP$_{escalated}$ might be too short; however, an even longer follow-up is needed. It can be assumed that the reduction of radiotherapy to only every tenth patient might result in a markedly decreased risk of second solid tumors, which is also true for cardiovascular disease.[15]

CHALLENGES IN THE TREATMENT OF OLDER PATIENTS WITH INTENSIFIED REGIMENS

In patients older than 60 years, the dose density that is decisive for the success of early intensification treatment in HL often cannot be achieved because of intolerability. The type of toxicity does not differ significantly from that seen in younger patients. It generally involves leukopenia, infections, and cardiopulmonary events.[16–19] However, these side effects are usually much more severe and a considerable percentage of patients older than 60 years dies of acute TRM.[17] As the most common cause of death during treatment is infection, it was hoped that the use of G-CSF would reduce the number of severe events. There are no specific studies for answering this question in HL, but in elderly non-HL patients this hypothesis has not been confirmed.[20,21] In patients older than 60 years, results with BEACOPP$_{escalated}$ have been poor. In the age group between 60 and 65 years, treatment-associated mortality was 14% and hence in the follow-up studies an age limit of 60 years was set, meaning that dose intensification might not be feasible in elderly patients in contrast to younger patients and thus might not improve the outcome. Unfortunately, this hypothesis has been confirmed in clinical trials performed by the GHSG. These studies investigated BEACOPP-derived regimens and did not have a positive outcome. In the HD9 Elderly Study, COPP/ABVD was compared with 8 cycles of BEACOPP$_{baseline}$, with only 55% of patients able to receive the intended number of cycles of BEACOPP$_{baseline}$. Disease-specific survival after 5 years was much better for the aggressive BEACOPP regimen (74% vs 55%), but this benefit did not translate into improved OS after 5 years because of the large number of treatment-associated deaths in the BEACOPP arm (21% vs 8% compared with COPP/ABVD).[18] It was thought that the etoposide in the BEACOPP regimen contributed to the poor tolerability in this population and it was therefore omitted in the follow-up study (BACOPP).[22] In this study, the complete remission rate was high (85%) but 87% of patients suffered grade III/IV toxicity and after a median follow-up of just 3 years there were 18 deaths of a total population of 60 patients (30%). There were 7 treatment-associated deaths among them, which corresponds to 12%. Treatment-associated mortality of 10% or more is not considered acceptable and the early intensification treatment approach for older patients has been abandoned by the GHSG. ABVD as a presumably better tolerated regimen cannot be recommended for this patient population as well because of unacceptable lung toxicity and poor overall tolerability.[23,24] Acute TRM in the most recent study with ABVD was 9%.[23,24] Current GHSG studies therefore investigate the implementation of noncytotoxic drugs within well-known chemotherapy backbones (ie, immunomodulation with lenalidomide in combination with AVD [doxorubicin, vinblastine, dacarbazine, lenalidomide]), or the anti-CD30 targeted drug brentuximab vedotin in combination with CHP (B-CAP: brentuximab vedotin, cyclophosphamide, doxorubicin, prednisone). The latter regimen will be investigated in cooperation with the Nordic Lymphoma Group.

EARLY OR LATE INTENSIFICATION? PROS AND CONS

Actually, which toxicities HL patients would accept to get the highest chance of cure has never been investigated. However, it seems unlikely that HL patients are very different from other patients with cancer. It is well known that patients with cancer are ready to accept intensive chemotherapies and its sequelae for only 1% survival benefit.[25] A well-performed survey in early-stage HL survivors showed that 80% of the patients consider relapse of HL as 1 of 3 most important potential problems.[14] Only development of second neoplasia was more important (88%). Interestingly, only 25% of patients ranked infertility as 1 of 3 most important potential problems. The general experience with the many thousands of patients treated in the 6 generations of the GHSG studies, men and women, echoes these published data and priorities for young patients confronted with a life-threatening disease and primarily wanting to be cured and to get back to a normal life as soon as possible. Given a 10% survival benefit for BEACOPP$_{escalated}$ at 5 years (**Fig. 1**) compared with initial treatment with ABVD, it is hard to imagine any good reason not to pursue this obviously superior regimen.[10,26]

Physicians advocating ABVD and the late intensification approach argue that the survival at 5 years is the same and the overall amount of toxicity is less, because 70% of patients are cured with ABVD alone and 30% need salvage therapy with high-dose chemotherapy and autologous stem cell support.[1]

Assuming a comparable OS (which has been shown not to be the case),[26] a 30% relapse rate is accepted by those advocating ABVD, which is 3-fold and thus a large increase in the risk of relapse compared indirectly with 6 cycles of BEACOPP$_{escalated}$. In addition, ABVD was significantly inferior in terms of PFS in all direct comparisons with BEACOPP variants (**Table 1**). Again, relapse is a very serious concern of HL patients even years after successful treatment, ranking far above infertility.[14] If physicians then accept relapses and high-dose chemotherapy for a third of all patients and recommend ABVD as first-line therapy, then one would expect to see also a really large benefit in terms of a less toxicities. However, which benefit does first-line treatment with ABVD offer?

Regarding randomized trials to assure comparability in terms of patient characteristics and treatment settings, there is no difference at all looking at the most feared events as second neoplasia, second AML/MDS, or acute TRM (**Table 2**).[27–30] Interestingly, even in the meta-analysis including more than 11,000 patients, events for TRM

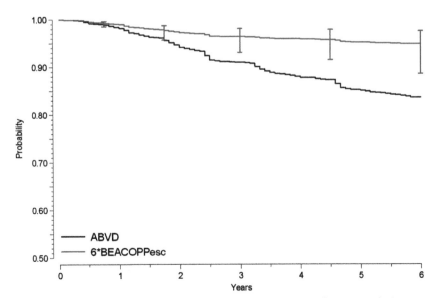

Fig. 1. OS of ABVD versus 6 cycles of BEACOPP$_{escalated}$ in a network meta-analysis.

Table 1
PFS and OS of ABVD and BEACOPP variants in all trials directly comparing these 2 different approaches (bottom line: 6 cycles of BEACOPP_escalated as standard of care)

Study	Group	N	5-y PFS	Difference in Favor of BEACOPP (%)	P	5-y OS	Difference in Favor of BEACOPP (%)
HD 2000[28]	ABVD	99	68	13	.038	84	8
	BEACOPP (4 esc + 2 std)	98	81			92	
IIL[27,a]	ABVD	168	73	12	.004	84	5
	BEACOPP (4 esc + 4 std)	163	85			89	
IG 20012[29,b]	ABVD	275	69	15	.0003	86.7	4
	BEACOPP (4 esc + 4 std)	274	84			90.3	
LYSA H34[30] IPS 1-3	ABVD	77	75	18	.008	92	7
	BEACOPP (4 esc + 4 std)	68	93			99	
HD15[8]	6 BEACOPPesc	711	91	—	—	95.3	—

Abbreviations: esc, escalated; std, standard.
[a] 7-year PFS and OS.
[b] 4-year PFS and OS.

or second neoplasia were too rare to allow for testing.[26] Obviously, longer follow-up is needed to help elucidate these questions. Until then, the existing evidence should be applied and irrational arguments that neither help doctors nor patients should be avoided.[4]

There certainly is a significant difference in terms of acute toxicities, especially regarding hematotoxicity. Whenever the health care setting is not suited to manage acute toxicities of BEACOPP_escalated adequately, ABVD might be applied as the second best choice.

Finally, gonadal toxicity is more pronounced with the early intensification approach as compared with those 70% of patients who are cured with ABVD only. For the third

Table 2
Relevant long-term toxicities of ABVD and BEACOPP variants in all trials directly comparing these 2 different approaches (bottom line: 6 cycles of BEACOPP_escalated as standard of care)

Study	Group	n	TRM (%)	sAML/MDS (%)	Second Neoplasia, n (%)
HD 2000[28]	ABVD	99	NR	0	1 (1)
	BEACOPP (4 esc + 2 std)	98	NR	0	1 (1)
IIL[27]	ABVD	168	1	1	3 (7.7)
	BEACOPP (4 esc + 4 std)	163	3	1	1 (0.6)
IG 20012[29]	ABVD	275	3.3	0.7	8 (2.9)
	BEACOPP (4 esc + 4 std)	274	2.2	1.5	10 (3.7)
LYSA H34[30] IPS 1-3	ABVD	77	0	0	5 (6.5)
	BEACOPP (4 esc + 4 std)	68	0	0	1 (1.5)
HD15[8]	6 BEACOPPesc	711	0.8	0.3	15 (2.1)

Abbreviation: NR, not reported.

of patients in need of salvage treatment including high-dose chemotherapy after ABVD failure, infertility (and severe hypogonadism in women) is obligatory, however. Nonetheless, in terms of relevant toxicities, gonadal damage is a disadvantage of the early intensification approach for most patients. The relative importance of this specific toxicity as compared with the importance of definite tumor control can differ extremely between individual patients. Treating physicians should provide the information on the efficacy and toxicity of the different treatment options to our patients. The patient can then choose best for his or her individual situation.

In summary, even if it is presumed that a comparable OS with the 2 different approaches, there is no good reason to recommend ABVD as first-line treatment. Definite tumor control with the primary treatment can undoubtedly be reached much better with BEACOPP$_{escalated}$ without an excess of meaningful toxicity (see **Tables 1** and **2**). In contrast to popular belief there is no difference in terms of TRM or second neoplasia compared with ABVD as has been documented in several studies (see **Table 2**). BEACOPP$_{escalated}$ can be easily managed even in primary care cancer centers. Regarding gonadal toxicity, the relative importance of this specific side effect as compared with the importance of being cured with the first-line treatment must be judged by the patient. In summary, there is no benefit of primary treatment with ABVD that could outweigh a 3-fold inferior PFS.

Finally, when discussing and setting the standard of care, it should be kept in mind why patients seek expertise and advice: they want to be cured from their malignant and life-threatening disease. Thus, OS remains the most relevant endpoint for the definition of a standard of care. As a matter of fact, OS is significantly and meaningfully better with BEACOPP$_{escalated}$ than with ABVD. Individual priorities might result in different individual treatment decisions; however, primary treatment recommendations should be based on evidence derived from clinical research. Referring to evidence-based knowledge, the early intensification approach with BEACOPP$_{escalated}$ must be called standard of care for advanced-stage HL patients.

REFERENCES

1. Connors JM. Hodgkin's lymphoma–the great teacher. N Engl J Med 2011;365(3): 264–5.
2. Diehl V, Franklin J, Pfreundschuh M, et al. Standard and increased-dose BEACOPP chemotherapy compared with COPP-ABVD for advanced Hodgkin's disease. N Engl J Med 2003;348(24):2386–95.
3. Borchmann P, Kreissl S, Diehl V, et al. Treatment of advanced-stage Hodgkin lymphoma: let us face the facts. J Clin Oncol 2013;31(24):3045–6.
4. Longo DL. Reply to P. Borchmann et al. J Clin Oncol 2013;31(24):3046.
5. Longo DL. Treatment of advanced hodgkin lymphoma: the more things change, the more they stay the same. J Clin Oncol 2013;31(6):660–2.
6. Engert A, Diehl V, Franklin J, et al. Escalated-dose BEACOPP in the treatment of patients with advanced-stage Hodgkin's lymphoma: 10 years of follow-up of the GHSG HD9 study. J Clin Oncol 2009;27:4548–54.
7. Borchmann P, Haverkamp H, Diehl V, et al. Eight cycles of escalated-dose BEACOPP compared with four cycles of escalated-dose BEACOPP followed by four cycles of baseline-dose BEACOPP with or without radiotherapy in patients with advanced-stage hodgkin's lymphoma: final analysis of the HD12 trial of the German Hodgkin Study Group. J Clin Oncol 2011;29(32):4234–42.
8. Engert A, Haverkamp H, Kobe C, et al. Reduced-intensity chemotherapy and PET-guided radiotherapy in patients with advanced stage Hodgkin's lymphoma

(HD15 trial): a randomised, open-label, phase 3 non-inferiority trial. Lancet 2012; 379(9828):1791–9.

9. Kobe C, Dietlein M, Franklin J, et al. Positron emission tomography has a high negative predictive value for progression or early relapse for patients with residual disease after first-line chemotherapy in advanced-stage Hodgkin lymphoma. Blood 2008;112(10):3989–94.

10. Andre M, Bosly A. BEACOPP escalated versus ABVD in advanced Hodgkin's lymphoma. Lancet Oncol 2013;14(10):911–2.

11. Wongso D, Fuchs M, Plutschow A, et al. Treatment-related mortality in patients with advanced-stage Hodgkin lymphoma: an analysis of the German Hodgkin study Group. J Clin Oncol 2013;31(22):2819–24.

12. Behringer K, Mueller H, Goergen H, et al. Gonadal function and fertility in survivors after Hodgkin lymphoma treatment within the German Hodgkin Study Group HD13 to HD15 trials. J Clin Oncol 2013;31(2):231–9.

13. Behringer K, Muller H, Gorgen H, et al. Sexual quality of life in Hodgkin Lymphoma: a longitudinal analysis by the German Hodgkin Study Group. Br J Cancer 2013;108(1):49–57.

14. Turner S, Maher EJ, Young T, et al. What are the information priorities for cancer patients involved in treatment decisions? An experienced surrogate study in Hodgkin's disease. Br J Cancer 1996;73(2):222–7.

15. Aleman BM, van den Belt-Dusebout AW, Klokman WJ, et al. Long-term cause-specific mortality of patients treated for Hodgkin's disease. J Clin Oncol 2003; 21(18):3431–9.

16. Engert A, Ballova V, Haverkamp H, et al. Hodgkin's lymphoma in elderly patients: a comprehensive retrospective analysis from the German Hodgkin's Study Group. J Clin Oncol 2005;23(22):5052–60.

17. Levis A, Depaoli L, Urgesi A, et al. Probability of cure in elderly Hodgkin's disease patients. Haematologica 1994;79(1):46–54.

18. Ballova V, Ruffer JU, Haverkamp H, et al. A prospectively randomized trial carried out by the German Hodgkin Study Group (GHSG) for elderly patients with advanced Hodgkin's disease comparing BEACOPP baseline and COPP-ABVD (study HD9 elderly). Ann Oncol 2005;16(1):124–31.

19. Enblad G, Glimelius B, Sundstrom C. Treatment outcome in Hodgkin's disease in patients above the age of 60: a population-based study. Ann Oncol 1991;2(4):297–302.

20. Bohlius J, Reiser M, Schwarzer G, et al. Impact of granulocyte colony-stimulating factor (CSF) and granulocyte-macrophage CSF in patients with malignant lymphoma: a systematic review. Br J Haematol 2003;122(3):413–23.

21. Doorduijn JK, van der Holt B, van Imhoff GW, et al. CHOP compared with CHOP plus granulocyte colony-stimulating factor in elderly patients with aggressive non-Hodgkin's lymphoma. J Clin Oncol 2003;21(16):3041–50.

22. Halbsguth TV, Nogova L, Mueller H, et al. Phase 2 study of BACOPP (bleomycin, adriamycin, cyclophosphamide, vincristine, procarbazine, and prednisone) in older patients with Hodgkin lymphoma: a report from the German Hodgkin Study Group (GHSG). Blood 2010;116(12):2026–32.

23. Proctor SJ, Wilkinson J, Jones G, et al. Evaluation of treatment outcome in 175 patients with Hodgkin lymphoma aged 60 years or over: the SHIELD study. Blood 2012;119(25):6005–15.

24. Evens AM, Hong F, Gordon LI, et al. The efficacy and tolerability of adriamycin, bleomycin, vinblastine, dacarbazine and Stanford V in older Hodgkin lymphoma patients: a comprehensive analysis from the North American intergroup trial E2496. Br J Haematol 2013;161(1):76–86.

25. Slevin ML, Stubbs L, Plant HJ, et al. Attitudes to chemotherapy: comparing views of patients with cancer with those of doctors, nurses, and general public. BMJ 1990;300(6737):1458–60.
26. Skoetz N, Trelle S, Rancea M, et al. Effect of initial treatment strategy on survival of patients with advanced-stage Hodgkin's lymphoma: a systematic review and network meta-analysis. Lancet Oncol 2013;14(10):943–52.
27. Viviani S, Zinzani PL, Rambaldi A, et al. ABVD versus BEACOPP for Hodgkin's lymphoma when high-dose salvage is planned. N Engl J Med 2011;365(3):203–12.
28. Federico M, Luminari S, Iannitto E, et al. ABVD compared with BEACOPP compared with CEC for the initial treatment of patients with advanced Hodgkin's lymphoma: results from the HD2000 Gruppo Italiano per lo Studio dei Linfomi Trial. J Clin Oncol 2009;27(5):805–11.
29. Carde P, Mounier N. ABVD (8 cycles) versus BEACOPP (4 escalated cycles ≥4 baseline) in stage III-IV high-risk Hodgkin lymphoma (HL): First results of EORTC 20012 Intergroup randomized phase III clinical trial. Annual Meeting of the Amercian Society of Clinical Oncology. Chicago, June 14–17, 2012. p. 8002.
30. Mounier N, Brice P, Bologna S, et al. ABVD (eight cycles) versus BEACOPP (4 escalated cycles to 4 baseline) in stages III-IV low risk Hodgkin lymphoma (IPS 0–2): final results of the LYSA H34 trial. Hematol Oncol 2013;31(Suppl 1):96–150 [abs 127].

Induction Therapy for Advanced-stage Hodgkin Lymphoma

Late Intensification (ABVD Chemotherapy Followed by High-dose Chemotherapy and Autologous Stem Cell Transplant Only for Those Who Relapse)

Stephen M. Ansell, MD, PhD

KEYWORDS

- Hodgkin lymphoma • ABVD chemotherapy • Escalated BEACOPP • Response rate
- Toxicity • Failure-free survival (FFS) • Event-free survival (EFS) • Overall survival (OS)

KEY POINTS

- Approximately 65% to 75% of advanced-stage Hodgkin lymphoma patients have a complete response to initial therapy with ABVD chemotherapy.
- The 5-year failure-free survival for advanced-stage Hodgkin lymphoma patients treated with ABVD is 70% to 75%.
- ABVD can be given to patients less than 60 years and patients with a poorer performance score.
- Although more intensive combinations, such as escalated BEACOPP, result in higher response rates and improved failure-free survival, the short- and long-term complications are greater.
- When all therapy including salvage therapy after initial treatment is considered, the outcomes of patients initially treated with ABVD or escalated BEACOPP were similar in a randomized trial. A network meta-analysis however showed a survival benefit with escalated BEACOPP.
- Because many patients are cured, exposing all patients to early intensive therapy increases the long-term complication risk in everyone. Reserving intensification for only those patients who need it decreases complications without clearly compromising overall outcome.

INTRODUCTION: NATURE OF THE PROBLEM

Hodgkin lymphoma is a B-cell malignancy that has been shown to be highly sensitive to chemotherapy.[1,2] The overall response rates to combination chemotherapy are in

Division of Hematology, Mayo Clinic, 200 First Street Southwest, Rochester, MN 55905, USA
E-mail address: ansell.stephen@mayo.edu

Hematol Oncol Clin N Am 28 (2014) 75–86
http://dx.doi.org/10.1016/j.hoc.2013.10.003
0889-8588/14/$ – see front matter © 2014 Elsevier Inc. All rights reserved.

excess of 70% and most patients are cured with standard therapy.[3] Patients with advanced-stage disease commonly have a higher risk of disease relapse than limited stage patients and often present with more poor prognostic features. Despite this, the percentage of patients who are cured by initial therapy is typically 70% to 75%.

ABVD chemotherapy (Adriamycin, Bleomycin, Vinblastine, and Dacarbazine) is a standard therapy for patients with Hodgkin lymphoma and is often used in North America to treat patients with advanced-stage disease. Typically patients receive 6 to 8 cycles of therapy, and provided they have had a complete response to the treatment that is PET negative, they will then be observed without further therapy. Some patients may have disease that proves to be resistant to this initial therapy and may require further treatment intensification. Other patients may subsequently relapse and then will receive salvage chemotherapy followed by high-dose chemotherapy with an autologous stem cell transplant.

A difference in opinion regarding optimal management of patients with advanced-stage Hodgkin lymphoma has developed over time. Some physicians think that an intensive approach as early as possible should be considered. Groups advocating this position commonly administer escalated BEACOPP (Bleomycin, Etoposide, Adriamycin, Cyclophosphamide, vincristine, Procarbazine, and Prednisone) chemotherapy for 6 cycles of treatment. They argue that an intensive approach will decrease the number of patients having an inadequate response to initial treatment and result in a greater percentage of patients who remain in remission and do not require further salvage chemotherapy. However, the more intensive escalated BEACOPP approach may be associated with a greater frequency of initial toxicities and treatment-related mortality, and a greater prevalence of long-term toxicities.

Those advocating for initially treating patients with less intense ABVD chemotherapy reason that the response rates are high with ABVD chemotherapy and the combination is substantially less toxic. ABVD chemotherapy can also be administered to older patients as well as those with a poor performance score at diagnosis, many of whom do not tolerate the more intensive approach. The minority of patients who fail this less intense initial treatment approach would then proceed to be treated in an intensive fashion with salvage chemotherapy followed by high-dose chemotherapy and an autologous stem cell transplant. Those physicians favoring the limited late intensification approach argue that most patients are not exposed to more intense chemotherapy and therefore the short-term and long-term complications are substantially less for most patients.

This concern about exposing all patients who generally have a very favorable prognosis to intensive therapy is illustrated by a study by Biasoli and colleagues[4] that looked at a Groupe d'Etudes des Lymphomes de l'Adulte/European Organisation for Research and Treatment of Cancer clinical trial randomizing patients between ABVD chemotherapy and escalated BEACOPP. They found that only one-half of the patients that were considered for the study at one of the participating centers were enrolled. The remaining patients chose not to participate. The choice not to participate was due to both patient and physician concerns. The main reason for patient's refusal was that they preferred the standard treatment (ABVD chemotherapy) and were concerned about toxicity in the experimental arm (escalated BEACOPP). When questioned further, the patient's main concern was the high incidence of anticipated infertility in the BEACOPP arm. Similarly, physicians chose not to enroll patients in the study because of their concerns with increased toxicity in the escalated BEACOPP arm. Subsequent studies by this group however have used escalated BEACOPP as initial therapy, suggesting that these attitudes may have changed over time.

CLINICAL OUTCOMES
Overall Results with ABVD Chemotherapy

Most patients have an excellent outcome after treatment with ABVD chemotherapy. Multiple studies evaluating the efficacy of ABVD chemotherapy have shown that on average 65% to 75% of advanced-stage Hodgkin lymphoma patients have a complete response to initial therapy with ABVD chemotherapy.[5-9] Studies that have evaluated interim positron emission tomography (PET) scans have shown approximately 75% of patients to be PET-negative after 2 to 3 cycles of ABVD chemotherapy, further confirming the high response rate. The 5-year failure-free survival for advanced-stage Hodgkin lymphoma treated with ABVD chemotherapy in multiple studies has been shown to be 70% to 75%. The following studies confirm the above-mentioned results:

- In the recently reported Eastern Cooperative Oncology Group clinical trial of ABVD chemotherapy compared with Stanford V chemotherapy (E2496),[5] 854 patients were treated and 395 of these patients received ABVD chemotherapy. The complete response rate for those receiving ABVD chemotherapy was 73% and the 5-year failure-free survival was 67% for advanced-stage patients receiving ABVD.
- In the HD9601 trial,[6] ABVD chemotherapy was compared with an intensive combination approach as well as with Stanford V chemotherapy. The 122 patients who received ABVD chemotherapy had a complete response rate of 89%. With long-term follow-up, the 5-year failure-free survival was 78% and the 10-year failure-free survival was 75%, suggesting that most of the patients that achieved a complete remission remained in remission and that approximately three-quarters of the patients were cured.
- In a randomized trial comparing ABVD chemotherapy with escalated BEACOPP chemotherapy conducted by Viviani and colleagues,[7] 331 patients were treated in the study, 166 of whom received ABVD chemotherapy. In this study, the complete response rate for ABVD-treated patients was 64% with a 73% 7-year failure-free survival.
- Similar results were seen in the HD2000 trial published by Federico and colleagues.[8] In this study, 307 patients were treated with escalated BEACOPP, an intensive combination chemotherapy regimen (cyclophosphamide, lomustine, vindesine, melphalan, prednisone, epidoxirubicin, vincristine, procarbazine, vinblastine, and bleomycin [COPPEBVCAD; CEC]), or ABVD chemotherapy. When the ABVD-treated patients are considered, the 103 patients who received ABVD chemotherapy had a complete response rate of 70% and a 5-year failure-free survival of 65%.
- Finally, in a United Kingdom study (ISRCTN64141244),[9] 520 patients were treated with either ABVD chemotherapy or Stanford V chemotherapy. Again, a complete response rate of 67% was seen in the 252 patients receiving the ABVD chemotherapy and the 5-year progression-free survival was 76%.

All of these studies suggest that approximately three-quarters of the patients treated with ABVD chemotherapy for advanced-stage Hodgkin lymphoma have a durable remission and are potentially cured with this approach.

Results with ABVD Compared with More Dose-intense Initial Therapy

Although the clinical outcomes with ABVD chemotherapy have been very good, randomized controlled trials have shown that an early intensification approach using escalated BEACOPP results in higher response rates and an improved failure-free survival. Whether the overall survival of patients treated with escalated BEACOPP is significantly different to those treated with ABVD chemotherapy is controversial. Randomized trials have not clearly shown an overall survival advantage,[7] but a meta-analysis by the Cochrane Group has shown that BEACOPP-treated patients have a superior overall outcome.[10] However, the improved response rate and failure-free survival with escalated BEACOPP comes at the cost of increased toxicity and lower rates of salvage for those who relapse.

In the German Hodgkin Study Group (GHSG) HD9 trial,[11] the failure-free survival at 10 years was 64%, 70%, or 82%, with overall response rates of 75%, 80%, or 86%, for patients treated with either COPP alternating with ABVD (arm A), baseline BEACOPP (arm B), or escalated BEACOPP (arm C), respectively (P<.001). Similarly, in the study by Federico and colleagues,[8] complete response rates in patients receiving ABVD chemotherapy, escalated BEACOPP chemotherapy, or the CEC regimen were 70%, 81%, and 69%, respectively. The 5-year failure-free survival in the ABVD chemotherapy-treated patients was 65% compared with 78% for those receiving escalated BEACOPP (P = .036), suggesting that response to treatment and durability of response may be improved in those receiving escalated BEACOPP.

However, to truly appreciate the merits of using an intensification approach early in all patients, or later only in relapsing patients, the outcome of all therapy needs to be considered, meaning that initial therapy and subsequent salvage approaches should be considered. In a recent randomized comparison of ABVD chemotherapy versus escalated BEACOPP,[7] 107 patients assigned to the ABVD chemotherapy group (64%) and 114 patients assigned to the escalated BEACOPP therapy (70%) had a complete response to initial therapy. The estimated 7-year rate of freedom from first progression in this population was 85% in the BEACOPP group as compared with 73% in the ABVD group, which was a significant difference of 12 percentage points (P = .004). However, when discontinuation of treatment owing to life-threatening toxic effects or secondary leukemias was considered, the difference of 7 percentage points between the 7-year event free-survival rate (78%) in those receiving BEACOPP versus 71% in those receiving ABVD failed to reach significance (P = .15). When the 65 patients who did not have a complete response to initial therapy or who subsequently relapsed were considered, there were 45 in the ABVD-treated group and 20 patients in the escalated BEACOPP group. Two-thirds of the patients in both groups could receive high-dose consolidation chemotherapy that included high-dose treatment followed by an autologous stem cell transplant. A similar percentage of patients in both groups were unable to start salvage treatment or did not complete the salvage regimen due to poor performance score or progressive disease. The complete response rate at the end of salvage treatment was higher among those who had initially received ABVD chemotherapy than among those who had initially received escalated BEACOPP (51% vs 35%). Of the patients who received ABVD chemotherapy, 33% remained alive and free of disease after salvage treatment compared with 15% in the escalated BEACOPP group. After completion of all of the assigned treatment in the study including subsequent salvage therapy for those required it, the estimated 7-year rate of freedom from second progression was not significantly different—88% in the escalated BEACOPP group compared with 82% in the ABVD group (P = .12). The difference in the estimated 7-year overall survival rate (89% in the escalated BEACOPP group compared with 84% in the ABVD group) was also not statistically significant (P = .39). However, it should be noted that this trial has been criticized for being underpowered to detect a difference in overall outcome.

Overall, escalated BEACOPP chemotherapy does induce a greater percentage of patients to achieve a complete remission and results in a higher percentage of patients who remain free from disease progression after initial therapy. However, when salvage therapy is also considered (initial therapy plus an autologous transplant if patients have resistant or progressive disease), patients who initially receive ABVD chemotherapy have a similarly favorable overall outcome to those who initially received escalated BEACOPP therapy.[7] The overall outcome after all therapy shows a similar failure-free survival after second therapy and a similar overall survival. The main consideration therefore is whether all patients should be treated with an intensive chemotherapy approach or whether it is preferable to administer a more modest treatment initially for the three-quarters of patients that will be cured by this treatment and only expose a quarter of patients to late intensified treatment, thereby significantly minimizing the side effects of treatment.

Results with Subsequent Salvage Chemotherapy After Initial ABVD Chemotherapy

Although it could be argued that the "first shot is the best and only shot," data would suggest that most patients who have subsequent disease progression after ABVD can be successfully salvaged with a late intensification approach. In a retrospective review of their treatment strategy, Gallamini and colleagues[12] treated patients with ABVD chemotherapy for 2 cycles with the plan to escalate treatment to BEACOPP if a PET scan during therapy was abnormal due to persistent disease. In this review, most patients did very well with ABVD chemotherapy and 83% of the 155 patients treated had a negative interim PET scan. Most patients who were PET2-negative remained in remission and the 2-year failure-free survival of PET2-negative patients was 92%. Only 23 patients had an abnormal interim PET scan and required escalated BEACOPP treatment. Of these patients, 15 achieved a continuous complete remission confirming that initial treatment with ABVD did not significantly compromise the likelihood of a response to subsequent intensification.

In a separate study by Wannesson and colleagues,[13] salvage chemotherapy with an autologous stem cell transplant after initial treatment was studied. Patients who initially received ABVD chemotherapy had a greater likelihood of successful salvage therapy than those who received escalated BEACOPP. When the chemosensitive Hodgkin lymphoma patients autografted after failure of escalated BEACOPP (n = 22) were compared with 22 cases of those who received a salvage autologous transplant after ABVD chemotherapy, the 5-year progression-free survival was 76% for ABVD-treated patients and 42% for those who received escalated BEACOPP ($P = .029$). These data would suggest that patients who relapse after ABVD chemotherapy can successfully be salvaged in most cases with an autologous stem cell transplant.

COMPLICATIONS AND CONCERNS
Acute Toxicity

Hematologic toxicity

Although ABVD chemotherapy does induce hematological toxicity, the combination can be safely administered to most patients less than 60 years of age. In an analysis of 1182 younger patients (<60 years) by Böll and colleagues,[14] only 7.5% of young patients had grade 3 or 4 leucopenia with 4 cycles of ABVD chemotherapy. Even elderly patients (>60 years, n = 117) could tolerate the regimen reasonably well with grade 3 or 4 leucopenia seen in 42% of older patients but 86% of elderly patients receiving all treatment as per protocol. More intensive approaches including escalated BEACOPP, in contrast, have significant short-term acute complications, particularly hematologic toxicity, and are typically given to patients less than 60 years.

Various supportive therapies are needed when intensive combinations such as escalated BEACOPP are administered. Engert and colleagues[15] reported a study of patients who received erythropoietin versus placebo as a way to manage the red cell transfusions required in patients receiving escalated BEACOPP. Although they found in this study that the median number of red cell transfusions was reduced from 4 per patient in those receiving placebo to 2 per patient for those receiving erythropoietin, it was notable that only 24.4% of patients required no red cell transfusions while receiving the escalated BEACOPP combination.

A further study by Borchmann and colleagues[16] reported on significant acute toxicities including hematological toxicities associated with 8 cycles of escalated BEACOPP. In this study, 8 cycles of escalated BEACOPP was compared with 4 cycles of escalated BEACOPP followed by 4 cycles of baseline BEACOPP. Deaths related to acute toxicity from chemotherapy were observed in 2.9% of patients receiving escalated BEACOPP chemotherapy. The reduction to the 4 plus 4 regimen did not significantly reduce the severe toxicity but seemed to potentially compromise efficacy.

Infection

Severe infections in patients treated with ABVD are uncommon even when full doses of treatment are given as scheduled despite the presence of neutropenia.[17] Similar results were seen in an analysis of 1167 patients less than age 60 treated with ABVD,[14] in whom only 4% had grade 3 or 4 infection. However, the difference in infection risk between those receiving ABVD chemotherapy and escalated BEACOPP seems substantial. In the HD9 trial,[11] 3 patients died of infection in those treated with ABVD chemotherapy compared with 22 patients who received escalated BEACOPP. In the study by Federico and colleagues,[8] 2 patients receiving ABVD chemotherapy had grade 3 to 4 infections compared with 14 patients who received escalated BEACOPP.

Treatment-related mortality

Deaths while on treatment are always a concern and may be increased in patients treated with an early intensification approach. In the trial by Viviani and colleagues,[7] 1 of the 168 patients treated with ABVD chemotherapy died on treatment compared with 5 of 163 patients treated with escalated BEACOPP. A difference in treatment-related mortality was not seen however in the EORTC/GELA 20012 trial, and 6 toxic deaths occurred in the 275 ABVD-treated patients compared with 5 toxic deaths in the 274 patients treated with 4 escalated BEACOPP and 4 cycles of baseline BEACOPP.[18] In an analysis of 3402 patients treated with escalated BEACOPP recently reported by Wongso and colleagues,[19] the treatment-related mortality seen with escalated BEACOPP was 1.9%. It was notable, however, that most patients in this study were less than 60 years of age. When those older than 50 years of age were analyzed, the treatment-related mortality increased to 5.7%. Even when those older than 40 years of age were considered, patients in this age group with a poor performance score (2 or greater) had a dramatically increased risk of treatment-related mortality of 15%. These data suggest that the risk of treatment-related mortality may be higher with early intensification than with a late intensification approach using high-dose chemotherapy and an autologous stem cell transplant[20] and supports limiting intensification strategies to only those patients who really need it.

In acknowledgment of the treatment-related mortality associated with an early escalation approach for all patients, the GHSG has looked at decreasing toxicity by decreasing the number of cycles of therapy given.[21] They found that 6 cycles of escalated BEACOPP showed similar results to 8 cycles of escalated BEACOPP with less toxicity. The 8-cycle group had a higher mortality (7.5%) than that seen with 6 cycles of escalated BEACOPP (4.6%) or with BEACOPP given on a 14-day schedule (5.2%). The main differences seen were in treatment-related events (2.1%) for 8 cycles of escalated BEACOPP compared with 0.8% for 6 cycles of escalated BEACOPP. Also noted were secondary malignancies, which were 1.8% in the 8 cycles of escalated BEACOPP group compared with 1.1% in the 6 cycles of escalated BEACOPP group.

Long-Term Toxicity

Leukemia risk

Significant long-term toxicities are associated with intensification at any time in a patient's treatment course. Therefore limiting the intensification approach to only those patients who clearly need it would be of significant benefit for them by decreasing the risk of long-term complications.

Acute myeloid leukemia is a known complication of an intensive treatment approach. Scholz and colleagues[22] showed that the cumulative risk of developing Acute myeloid leukemia was 1.5% for patients treated with chemotherapy (including ABVD) for advanced-stage Hodgkin lymphoma. In contrast, the risk of developing leukemia was increased after escalated BEACOPP and was 4.4% ($P = .004$). The risk of leukemia after escalated BEACOPP was comparable with that after treatment for relapse, which included an autologous stem cell transplant, which was 4.5%, suggesting that the leukemia risk associated with escalated BEACOPP seems similar to the leukemia risk with chemotherapy followed by an autologous stem cell transplant. Therefore limiting the number of patients who receive the intensification approach would be beneficial.

The high risk of second malignancies, including acute leukemia, has been seen in several clinical trials. In the HD9 trial[11] with 10 years of follow-up, a total of 74 second malignancies have been documented including acute myeloid leukemia in 0.4% of patients. In the HD12 trial,[16] there were 76 secondary malignancies (4.8%), and of these patients 22 had acute myeloid leukemia, 38 patients had solid tumors, and 16 patients developed non-Hodgkin lymphoma.

Infertility

A significant concern with intensified therapy is loss of fertility. ABVD chemotherapy was specifically designed to preserve fertility and the rate of long-term infertility after ABVD chemotherapy is less than 10%.[23–25] Overall, approximately one-third of male patients develop transient azoospermia after ABVD chemotherapy, and almost no female patients experience ovarian failure.[26]

Because treatment has been escalated, the risk of infertility has become substantially greater. Strategies to prevent infertility have been attempted but it has proven challenging to prevent infertility with more intensive treatment. In women receiving escalated BEACOPP, Behringer and colleagues[27] showed that infertility could not be prevented. The GHSG investigated the use of gonadotropin-releasing hormone analogues and oral contraceptives as a strategy to prevent infertility in young women with advanced Hodgkin lymphoma receiving escalated BEACOPP. For the entire group of patients, the ovarian follicle preservation rate was 0%.[27] A subsequent study by Behringer and colleagues[28] showed that after 6 to 8 cycles of escalated BEACOPP, 45% of patients ceased menstrual activity if they were older than 30 years of age and the time to recovery of the menstrual cycle was also prolonged with higher dose chemotherapy. Thirty-four percent of women older than 30 years suffered severe menopausal symptoms, which was 3 to 4 times more frequent than expected.

In men, fertility is further compromised by the fact that many patients have low sperm counts secondary to the disease. In a pretreatment analysis (n = 202), 20% of patients had normozoospermia, 11% had azoospermia, and 69% had some other dyspermia.[29] However, similar to the study in women, Behringer and colleagues[28] found that 88% of male survivors after intensive treatment of advanced-stage Hodgkin lymphoma had oligospermia when inhibin B and follicle-stimulating hormone levels were evaluated. Furthermore, there was no recovery in inhibin B and follicle-stimulating hormone levels in any of these patients, indicating a lack of recovery of spermatogenesis, true for all patients who were survivors of advanced-stage Hodgkin lymphoma treated with BEACOPP on the HD15 trial. Interestingly, the levels of testosterone remained within the normal range after escalated BEACOPP, supporting the hypothesis that Leydig cells are more resistant to cytotoxic chemotherapy.

Stem cell injury
A further concern in patients treated with intensive treatment regimens is the increased risk of stem cell injury. In a study by Gobbi and colleagues,[30] ABVD chemotherapy had a very modest impact on stem cell function and was associated with the least early reduction and the best subsequent recovery of long-term culture-initiating cells when compared with other regimens. In contrast, escalated BEACOPP chemotherapy caused significantly greater early stem cell toxicity and this effect persisted for at least 6 months.

Cardiac toxicity
Cardiotoxicity is also a concern when patients receive chemotherapy combinations that include cardiotoxic agents such as doxorubicin. Both ABVD chemotherapy and BEACOPP chemotherapy contain doxorubicin and both combinations have demonstrated similar subclinical cardiotoxicity. Intensification of the therapy does not seem to impact cardiotoxicity as more intensive regimens such as escalated BEACOPP are not associated with a higher rate of cardiac impairment.[31]

Pulmonary toxicity
For patients receiving bleomycin, a drug that is present in both ABVD and BEACOPP, pulmonary toxicity is also a concern. Bleomycin lung toxicity is a potentially life-threatening complication and may be more prevalent in patients receiving ABVD chemotherapy. In a study by Martin and colleagues,[32] 27% of patients who received ABVD chemotherapy had bleomycin lung toxicity. In contrast, most studies evaluating escalated BEACOPP reported respiratory complications in 6% to 9% of patients[21] and deaths from bleomycin lung toxicity are rare.[16]

Toxicity in the elderly
An additional issue with using an early intensification approach is that older patients are unable to be treated with very aggressive therapy. In almost all of the studies using escalated BEACOPP as initial induction therapy, patients were not enrolled once they were older than 60 years of age. However, in a prospectively randomized study for older patients (HD9 elderly trial),[33] 75 patients aged 66 to 75 years with newly diagnosed advanced-stage Hodgkin lymphoma were enrolled to compare the BEACOPP regimen to COPP-ABVD. There were no significant differences between COPP-ABVD and BEACOPP in terms of complete remission (76%), overall survival (50%), or freedom from treatment failure (46%) at 5 years. However, toxicity between the regimens was quite different: 2 patients (8%) treated with COPP-ABVD compared with 9 patients (21%) treated with BEACOPP died of acute toxicity.

Other studies have confirmed the lower likelihood of toxicity when elderly patients are treated with ABVD. In an analysis of elderly patients (>60 years, n = 44) with advanced-stage Hodgkin lymphoma accrued to the North American intergroup trial E2496,[34] the overall treatment-related mortality for older patients receiving either ABVD or the Stanford V regimen was 9% compared with 0.3% for patients aged less than 60 years. Although the long-term outcome for older patients was not as good as for younger patients, the 5-year time to progression of 68% and 5-year overall survival of 58% was acceptable in this high-risk population. These results suggest that ABVD chemotherapy may be a better choice than intensive regimens as initial therapy for elderly patients with advanced Hodgkin lymphoma.

SUMMARY

ABVD chemotherapy remains an effective combination for patients with advanced-stage Hodgkin lymphoma and approximately 65% to 75% of patients who receive ABVD chemotherapy for advanced-stage disease have a complete response to initial treatment. Studies using PET scans have confirmed that three-quarters of patients have a complete response to treatment and these responses seem durable. To confirm this further, the 5-year failure-free survival for advanced age Hodgkin lymphoma patients treated with ABVD chemotherapy is typically 70% to 75%. ABVD chemotherapy can generally be administered to patients who typically have had a poorer prognosis, including patients over 60 years of age and patients who initially present with a poor performance score. In contrast, intensified treatment approaches, including escalated BEACOPP, are unsuitable for these patients as the likelihood of treatment-related toxicity is dramatically higher.

Although intensive combinations including escalated BEACOPP have been shown in randomized trials to result in a higher overall response rate and an improved failure-free survival, this benefit is commonly offset by both short-term and long-term complications. An early intensification approach typically has resulted in a greater number of patients with infectious complications. Furthermore, a greater percentage of patients may subsequently develop secondary malignancies, including acute myeloid leukemia.

Patients who fail initial ABVD chemotherapy have been shown to respond to salvage chemotherapy. Typical salvage chemotherapy is followed by a high-dose therapy with an autologous stem cell transplant, and the likelihood of responding to this approach is greater for those who initially received ABVD chemotherapy than for those who underwent an early intensification approach. When salvage chemotherapy after initial treatment is included in the survival analysis, the outcomes of patients who are initially treated with ABVD chemotherapy or with an intensification approach are similar. When all patients treated with ABVD chemotherapy, and subsequently an autologous stem cell transplant for the subset who relapse, are compared with all patients who received escalated BEACOPP, including a transplant for the subset who progress, it is not clear that there is a significant overall survival outcome difference between the 2 groups.

Because many patients can be cured with ABVD chemotherapy, it may not be appropriate to expose all patients to early intensive therapy. As described above, approximately three-quarters of patients will be cured with ABVD chemotherapy. This regimen is well tolerated and has substantially less toxicity than escalated BEACOPP. In view of this fact, exposing all patients to an early intensified approach increases the long-term complication risk in all patients. It is therefore far more appropriate to reserve the intensification approach for only those patients who need it, this group being the minority of patients who are resistant to ABVD chemotherapy or who subsequently relapses. In this small subset of patients the increased risk of complications associated with intensified treatment is entirely justified.

Decreasing complications and improving long-term outcomes should be the goal of all therapy for patients with Hodgkin lymphoma. Therefore using an intensification approach only later in the disease course, and only in patients who clearly have shown they to need it decreases the overall long-term complications of therapy without substantially compromising outcomes. In the future, it is hoped that novel treatment combinations will increase efficacy and decrease toxicity, thereby improving the survival of Hodgkin lymphoma patients.

REFERENCES

1. Kanzler H, Kuppers R, Hansmann ML, et al. Hodgkin and Reed-Sternberg cells in Hodgkin's disease represent the outgrowth of a dominant tumor clone derived from (crippled) germinal center B cells. J Exp Med 1996;184:1495–505.
2. Marafioti T, Hummel M, Foss HD, et al. Hodgkin and Reed-Sternberg cells represent an expansion of a single clone originating from a germinal center B-cell with functional immunoglobulin gene rearrangements but defective immunoglobulin transcription. Blood 2000;95:1443–50.
3. Ansell SM. Hodgkin lymphoma: 2012 update on diagnosis, risk-stratification, and management. Am J Hematol 2012;87(12):1096–103.
4. Biasoli I, Franchi-Rezgui P, Sibon D, et al. Analysis of factors influencing inclusion of 102 patients with stage III/IV Hodgkin's lymphoma in a randomized trial for first-line chemotherapy. Ann Oncol 2008;19(11):1915–20.
5. Gordon LI, Hong F, Fisher RI, et al. Randomized phase III trial of ABVD versus Stanford V with or without radiation therapy in locally extensive and advanced-stage Hodgkin lymphoma: an intergroup study coordinated by the Eastern Cooperative Oncology Group (E2496). J Clin Oncol 2013;31(6):684–91.
6. Chisesi T, Bellei M, Luminari S, et al. Long-term follow-up analysis of HD9601 trial comparing ABVD versus Stanford V versus MOPP/EBV/CAD in patients with newly diagnosed advanced-stage Hodgkin's lymphoma: a study from the Intergruppo Italiano Linfomi. J Clin Oncol 2011;29(32):4227–33.
7. Viviani S, Zinzani PL, Rambaldi A, et al. ABVD versus BEACOPP for Hodgkin's lymphoma when high-dose salvage is planned. N Engl J Med 2011;365:203–12.
8. Federico M, Luminari S, Iannitto E, et al. ABVD compared with BEACOPP compared with CEC for the initial treatment of patients with advanced Hodgkin's lymphoma: results from the HD2000 Gruppo Italiano per lo Studio dei Linfomi Trial. J Clin Oncol 2009;27(5):805–11.
9. Hoskin PJ, Lowry L, Horwich A, et al. Randomized comparison of the stanford V regimen and ABVD in the treatment of advanced Hodgkin's Lymphoma: United Kingdom National Cancer Research Institute Lymphoma Group Study ISRCTN 64141244. J Clin Oncol 2009;27(32):5390–6.
10. Skoetz N, Trelle S, Rancea M, et al. Effect of initial treatment strategy on survival of patients with advanced-stage Hodgkin's lymphoma: a systematic review and network meta-analysis. Lancet Oncol 2013;14(10):943–52.
11. Engert A, Diehl V, Franklin J, et al. Escalated-dose BEACOPP in the treatment of patients with advanced-stage Hodgkin's lymphoma: 10 years of follow-up of the GHSG HD9 study. J Clin Oncol 2009;27(27):4548–54.
12. Gallamini A, Patti C, Viviani S, et al. Early chemotherapy intensification with BEACOPP in advanced-stage Hodgkin lymphoma patients with a interim-PET positive after two ABVD courses. Br J Haematol 2011;152(5):551–60.
13. Wannesson L, Bargetzi M, Cairoli A, et al. Autotransplant for Hodgkin lymphoma after failure of upfront BEACOPP escalated (bleomycin, etoposide, doxorubicin, cyclophosphamide, vincristine, procarbazine and prednisone). Leuk Lymphoma 2013;54(1):36–40.

14. Böll B, Görgen H, Fuchs M, et al. ABVD in older patients with early-stage Hodgkin lymphoma treated within the German Hodgkin Study Group HD10 and HD11 trials. J Clin Oncol 2013;31(12):1522–9.
15. Engert A, Josting A, Haverkamp H, et al. Epoetin alfa in patients with advanced-stage Hodgkin's lymphoma: results of the randomized placebo-controlled GHSG HD15EPO trial. J Clin Oncol 2010;28(13):2239–45.
16. Borchmann P, Haverkamp H, Diehl V, et al. Eight cycles of escalated-dose BEACOPP compared with four cycles of escalated-dose BEACOPP followed by four cycles of baseline-dose BEACOPP with or without radiotherapy in patients with advanced-stage Hodgkin's lymphoma: final analysis of the HD12 trial of the German Hodgkin Study Group. J Clin Oncol 2011;29(32):4234–42.
17. Evens AM, Cilley J, Ortiz T, et al. G-CSF is not necessary to maintain over 99% dose-intensity with ABVD in the treatment of Hodgkin lymphoma: low toxicity and excellent outcomes in a 10-year analysis. Br J Haematol 2007;137(6): 545–52.
18. Carde PP, Karrasch M, Fortpied C, et al. ABVD (8 cycles) versus BEACOPP (4 escalated cycles ≥4 baseline) in stage III-IV high-risk Hodgkin lymphoma (HL): first results of EORTC 20012 Intergroup randomized phase III clinical trial. J Clin Oncol 2012;30(Suppl) [abstract: 8002].
19. Wongso D, Fuchs M, Plütschow A, et al. Treatment-related mortality in patients with advanced-stage Hodgkin lymphoma: an analysis of the German Hodgkin Study Group. J Clin Oncol 2013;31(22):2819–24.
20. Majhail NS, Weisdorf DJ, Defor TE, et al. Long-term results of autologous stem cell transplantation for primary refractory or relapsed Hodgkin's lymphoma. Biol Blood Marrow Transplant 2006;12(10):1065–72.
21. Engert A, Haverkamp H, Kobe C, et al. Reduced-intensity chemotherapy and PET-guided radiotherapy in patients with advanced stage Hodgkin's lymphoma (HD15 trial): a randomised, open-label, phase 3 non-inferiority trial. Lancet 2012;379(9828):1791–9.
22. Scholz M, Engert A, Franklin J, et al. Impact of first- and second-line treatment for Hodgkin's lymphoma on the incidence of AML/MDS and NHL–experience of the German Hodgkin's Lymphoma Study Group analyzed by a parametric model of carcinogenesis. Ann Oncol 2011;22(3):681–8.
23. Harel S, Fermé C, Poirot C. Management of fertility in patients treated for Hodgkin's lymphoma. Haematologica 2011;96(11):1692–9.
24. Viviani S, Santoro A, Ragni G, et al. Gonadal toxicity after combination chemotherapy for Hodgkin's disease. Comparative results of MOPP vs ABVD. Eur J Cancer Clin Oncol 1985;21(5):601–5.
25. Kulkarni SS, Sastry PS, Saikia TK, et al. Gonadal function following ABVD therapy for Hodgkin's disease. Am J Clin Oncol 1997;20(4):354–7.
26. van der Kaaij MA, van Echten-Arends J, Simons AH, et al. Fertility preservation after chemotherapy for Hodgkin lymphoma. Hematol Oncol 2010;28(4): 168–79.
27. Behringer K, Wildt L, Mueller H, et al. No protection of the ovarian follicle pool with the use of GnRH-analogues or oral contraceptives in young women treated with escalated BEACOPP for advanced-stage Hodgkin lymphoma. Final results of a phase II trial from the German Hodgkin Study Group. Ann Oncol 2010;21(10): 2052–60.
28. Behringer K, Mueller H, Goergen H, et al. Gonadal function and fertility in survivors after Hodgkin lymphoma treatment within the German Hodgkin Study Group HD13 to HD15 trials. J Clin Oncol 2013;31(2):231–9.

29. Sieniawski M, Reineke T, Josting A, et al. Assessment of male fertility in patients with Hodgkin's lymphoma treated in the German Hodgkin Study Group (GHSG) clinical trials. Ann Oncol 2008;19(10):1795–801.

30. Gobbi PG, Rosti V, Valentino F, et al. The early- and intermediate-term toxicity to primitive hematopoietic progenitor cells of three chemotherapy regimens for advanced Hodgkin lymphoma. Clin Lymphoma Myeloma 2009;9(6):425–9.

31. Elbl L, Vasova I, Kral Z, et al. Evaluation of acute and early cardiotoxicity in survivors of Hodgkin's disease treated with ABVD or BEACOPP regimens. J Chemother 2006;18(2):199–208.

32. Martin WG, Ristow KM, Habermann TM, et al. Bleomycin pulmonary toxicity has a negative impact on the outcome of patients with Hodgkin's lymphoma. J Clin Oncol 2005;23(30):7614–20.

33. Ballova V, Rüffer JU, Haverkamp H, et al. A prospectively randomized trial carried out by the German Hodgkin Study Group (GHSG) for elderly patients with advanced Hodgkin's disease comparing BEACOPP baseline and COPP-ABVD (study HD9elderly). Ann Oncol 2005;16(1):124–31.

34. Evens AM, Hong F, Gordon LI, et al. The efficacy and tolerability of adriamycin, bleomycin, vinblastine, dacarbazine and Stanford V in older Hodgkin lymphoma patients: a comprehensive analysis from the North American intergroup trial E2496. Br J Haematol 2013;161(1):76–86.

FDG-PET Response–adapted Therapy
Is 18F-Fluorodeoxyglucose Positron Emission Tomography a Safe Predictor for a Change of Therapy?

Martin Hutchings, MD, PhD

KEYWORDS

- FDG-PET • PET/CT • Interim • Hodgkin • Lymphoma • Response adapted

KEY POINTS

- Fluorodeoxyglucose (FDG) positron emission tomography (PET) performed during or after chemotherapy is the strongest predictor of outcome in Hodgkin lymphoma.
- A large number of active trials have investigated the value of early PET response–adapted Hodgkin lymphoma therapy.
- Preliminary reports from recently completed trials are encouraging, but data are immature, and the use of PET response–adapted therapy is discouraged outside clinical trials.
- Postchemotherapy FDG-PET/computed tomography is a safe tool to identify advanced patients without the need for consolidation radiotherapy.
- Standardized image acquisition and image interpretation criteria are essential for the value and the use of interim FDG-PET.

INTRODUCTION
The Hodgkin Lymphoma Therapeutic Dilemma

The treatment of patients with Hodgkin lymphoma (HL) requires a delicate balance between high treatment efficacy and acceptable acute and late treatment-related toxicity. Overall long-term survival from HL exceeds 80% with modern therapy.[1] These excellent cure rates are a result of the high chemosensitivity and radiosensitivity of the disease, of the evolution of cytotoxic drugs and radiotherapy techniques but also of important developments in staging accuracy, identification of prognostic factors, and optimization of treatment according to well-defined risk groups. However, the

The author has no relevant disclosures.
Department of Haematology, Rigshospitalet, 9 Blegdamsvej, DK-2100 Copenhagen, Denmark
E-mail address: martin.hutchings@gmail.com

Hematol Oncol Clin N Am 28 (2014) 87–103
http://dx.doi.org/10.1016/j.hoc.2013.10.008
0889-8588/14/$ – see front matter © 2014 Elsevier Inc. All rights reserved.

efficacy of treatment is hampered by serious long-term adverse effects, including heart and lung disease, and secondary malignancies. As a consequence of these acute and late toxicities, patients with HL have an excessive mortality.[2] At 15 years following treatment, the risk of death from HL is overtaken by the risk of death from other causes.[3] The most important goal of contemporary clinical HL research is to address this problem and to optimize the balance between efficacy and toxicity. In order to reduce the long-term effects of treatment, therapeutic strategies are becoming more tailored to the individual patient's disease profile and other clinical characteristics. The aim is to maintain and improve the high cure rates while reducing therapy-related morbidity and mortality.[1]

Patients with early-stage disease have a chance of cure that exceeds 90% when treated with combined-modality treatment (ie, chemotherapy followed by radiotherapy to the initially involved lymph nodes or lymph node regions). With such high cure rates, it is more than likely that a substantial proportion of patients could be treated with less therapy than is currently considered standard practice. In the light of the serious long-term morbidity and mortality attributed to radiotherapy, it is desirable to identify the patients who might be cured with less treatment burden, particularly without radiotherapy.[4,5]

In advanced-stage disease, around two-thirds of patients can be cured with 6 to 8 cycles of the Adriamycin, bleomycin, vinblastine, and dacarbazine (ABVD) combination. Patients who have primary refractory disease or who relapse after first remission may be cured by high-dose salvage regimens, but 20% to 25% of ABVD-treated advanced-stage patients still die of treatment-resistant or relapsed HL.[6] In comparison, the more intensive and more toxic bleomycin, etoposide, doxorubicin, cyclophosphamide, vincristine, procarbazine, prednisone (BEACOPPesc) regimen yields significantly higher cure rates.[7] However, treating all patients with advanced-stage HL with BEACOPPesc means overtreatment of most patients, who would have been cured with ABVD.

However, the existing pretreatment prognostic scoring systems are not strongly predictive. There are therefore no pretreatment predictive markers to safely identify those patients who are more likely to be cured with less therapy on, and those patients who require more intensive treatment, both in early-stage and advanced-stage disease.

Fluorodeoxyglucose Positron Emission Tomography in HL

A more patient-tailored treatment may be achieved by more refined and risk-adapted selection of up-front therapy and by subsequent treatment modifications that reflect the individual patient's treatment sensitivity and response. The optimal up-front therapy selection demands precise determination of the initial disease extent, and, for this purpose, staging positron emission tomography (PET)/computed tomography (CT) has been accepted as the gold standard method in HL. Over the last 15 years, positron PET using 2-[18]fluoro-2-deoxyglucose (FDG) has gained widespread use in most lymphoma subtypes. Stand-alone FDG-PET has largely been replaced by combined scanners, in which FDG-PET and CT are performed in 1 scanning session, resulting in fusion PET/CT displaying pathologic anatomy and tumor physiology/metabolism in combined images. The European Society of Medical Oncology clinical practice guidelines and the National Comprehensive Cancer Network guidelines recommend the use of PET/CT for primary staging and final response evaluation in patients with HL.[8,9] Furthermore, it is generally agreed that the modern and highly conformal radiotherapy volumes that have become standard in HL are only safe when based on the most accurate baseline imaging (ie, PET/CT).[10]

After initiation of chemotherapy, and in the absence of strong pretreatment predictive markers, an early assessment of treatment sensitivity may allow identification of patients with low treatment sensitivity who might benefit from escalation to more aggressive therapy, and also of patients with high treatment sensitivity who could be cured with less than standard therapy. After completion of chemotherapy, a reliable response assessment is crucial to guide further management, including consolidation radiotherapy, follow-up, and salvage therapy in cases of refractory or relapsed disease.

Numerous studies have shown that PET/CT provides the most reliable assessment of chemosensitivity and response during and after completion of HL therapy.[11] As a result, the method plays an important role in current efforts to further optimize therapy. This article addresses the role of FDG-PET/CT for response-adapted HL therapy, both in the first-line setting and in relapsed disease.

EARLY TREATMENT MONITORING WITH FDG-PET

Clinical stage and prognostic factors are used to determine the initial treatment strategy for patients with HL. However, the tumor response to induction treatment is strongly prognostic. A reliable and early prediction of response to therapy may identify good-risk patients who will be cured with conventional therapy or even less intensive and less toxic regimens, and poor-risk patients for whom an early switch to alternative, more aggressive treatment strategies could improve the chance of remission and cure. This concept, called risk-adapted therapy, is a potential way to maintain or improve the high cure rates without increasing, and perhaps even decreasing, the risk of treatment-related morbidity and mortality.[12]

Conventional methods for treatment response monitoring are based on morphologic criteria, and a reduction in tumor size on CT is the most important determinant.[13] However, size reduction is not necessarily an accurate predictor of outcome. In HL, the malignant cells make up only a small fraction of the tumor volume, which is dominated by reactive infiltrating cells not directly affected by antineoplastic therapy.[14] Even more importantly, tumor shrinkage takes time and depends on several factors in the host. The rate of structural regression therefore cannot form the basis for therapy response assessment until late during treatment, at which point a treatment modification might be less useful.

As opposed to the morphologic changes of the lymphoma occurring later during therapy, functional imaging with FDG-PET enables early evaluation of the metabolic changes that take place early during the treatment induction. The rapid decrease in metabolic activity of cells in the tumor environment is highly predictive of the subsequent response and final outcome. Several studies of FDG-PET after 1 to 3 cycles of chemotherapy[15–20] have shown that these early metabolic changes are highly predictive of final treatment response and progression-free survival (PFS). Most evidence is available for FDG-PET after 2 cycles of chemotherapy. However, there are data to suggest that the prognostic accuracy is already high after only 1 cycle of chemotherapy.[21]

In 2005, a retrospective analysis of 88 patients scanned after 2 or 3 cycles of ABVD-like chemotherapy for HL showed a 5-year PFS of 39% in the PET-positive group compared with 92% in the PET-negative group.[16] These results were later confirmed in several prospective studies,[17–20,22] showing excellent outcomes for patients becoming PET negative after 2 cycles of chemotherapy (approximately 95% long-term PFS) and poor outcomes for early PET-positive patients. In patients with advanced disease, the high prognostic value of early FDG-PET seems to dilute the role of the widely accepted International Prognostic Index (IPS), which is based on pre-therapeutic factors.[19,20] The prognostic value of PET/CT in advanced HL was recently validated in an international study that showed 3-year failure-free survival of 28% and 95% for early PET-positive and early PET-negative patients, respectively.[23] In this validation study, the interobserver agreement was high between 6 independent PET/CT reviewers using the Deauville criteria for interim PET, which have become widely recognized.[24] Apart from giving reproducible results, the Deauville criteria are simple in use, thus it is hoped that their use in most of the recently opened PET response–adapted trials will enhance comparability between clinical trials and also enable a better translation of clinical trial results into clinical practice outside of trials. Recent data strongly suggest that the negative predictive value of FDG-PET may be even higher if the test is performed after 1 cycle of chemotherapy for HL.[25]

The positive predictive value of early FDG-PET may be lower in patients treated with the more dose-intensive regimens such as BEACOPPesc than in patients treated with ABVD.[26] Also, the positive predictive value is lower in patients with early-stage HL, probably because of both the inherently better prognosis for this patient group and because of the subsequent radiotherapy, which may in many early-stage patients overcome an insufficient chemotherapy response.[17,20,27,28] **Table 1** provides an overview of the studies showing the prognostic value of early interim FDG-PET in HL.

PET RESPONSE–ADAPTED HL THERAPY: EARLY-STAGE DISEASE

More than 90% of patients with early-stage HL are cured with standard therapy. However, the patients still have a greatly reduced life expectancy because of

Table 1							
Prognostic value of FDG-PET after 1 to 3 cycles of chemotherapy in HL							
	Cycles of Chemotherapy Before Interim PET		PET Positive		PET Negative		
Investigators, Ref #, Year		Patients	Total	Treatment Failure, n (%)	Total	Treatment Failure, n (%)	Follow-up (mo)
Hutchings et al,[16] 2005	2–3	85	13	8 (62)	72	4 (6)	6–125
Hutchings et al,[17] 2006[P]	2	77	16	11 (69)	61	3 (5)	2–41
Zinzani et al,[15] 2006[P]	2	40	8	7 (88)	32	1 (3)	12–27
Gallamini et al,[18] 2006[P]	2	108	20	18 (90)	88	3 (3)	2–47
Gallamini et al,[19] 2007[P]	2	260	50	43 (86)	210	10 (5)	4–62
Cerci et al,[20] 2010[P]	2	104	30	16 (53)	74	6 (8)	32–40
Zinzani et al,[22] 2012	2	304	53	40 (75)	251	20 (8)	6–100
Biggi et al,[23] 2013	2	260	45	33 (73)	215	12 (6)	12–96
Hutchings et al, 2013[P, U]	1	126	37	22 (59)	89	5 (6)	8–56

Abbreviations: P, prospective study; U, unpublished data, submitted for publication.

treatment-related illness including second cancers and cardiopulmonary disease. Patients with early-stage HL more often die from late effects of therapy than from the disease itself,[29] which suggests that a substantial number of patients with early-stage HL are subject to some amount of overtreatment, and it is the background for an ongoing effort to reduce the treatment burden while still maintaining or improving cure rates.

Two or 4 cycles of ABVD chemotherapy followed by involved-field radiotherapy (IFRT) or involved-node radiotherapy (INRT) is widely regarded as standard of care for early-stage HL,[30–32] although 6 cycles of ABVD seem to be comparable in safety and long-term cure rates.[33] Before the PET era, several studies suggested that selected patients could be safely managed with even less treatment. The German H10 trial for patients with early-stage HL without risk factors showed that 2 cycles of ABVD followed by 20-Gy IFRT is as effective as, and less toxic than, 4 cycles of ABVD followed by 30-Gy IFRT.[4] The National Cancer Institute of Canada (NCIC) and the Eastern Cooperative Oncology Group (ECOG) randomized 399 patients with early-stage HL to either combined-modality treatment or ABVD chemotherapy alone. In the chemotherapy-alone arm, patients who achieved a complete or unconfirmed complete remission after 2 cycles of ABVD received only 2 additional chemotherapy cycles. Despite this abbreviated chemotherapy, 95% of patients who received only 4 cycles of ABVD were free from progression after 5 years' follow-up. These studies, among others, have inspired researchers to propose that some patients with early-stage HL may be treated with even less therapy. In contrast, and particularly among patients with risk factors, cure rates leave room for improvement because approximately 15% of patients experience treatment failure with 4 cycles of ABVD plus 30-Gy INRT.[5] The German HD14 study showed that replacing 4 cycles of ABVD with 2 of BEACOPPesc followed by 2 of ABVD resulted in a small but significant 6 percentage-point benefit to PFS at 5 years.[34] This finding did not translate into an improved overall survival (OS), and most colleagues find it undesirable to offer intensified treatment to all patients with early unfavorable HL in order to gain improved outcome for very few patients. However, these studies have shown that one size does not fit all in early-stage HL. The high prognostic accuracy of the early interim FDG-PET makes the method a likely tool to guide early response–adapted therapy, aiming to improve management by minimizing therapy in most early-stage patients, who respond well, and perhaps intensifying therapy in a high-risk, poor-responding minority.

Several trials have assessed such PET response–adapted therapy for early-stage HL (**Table 2**). In the National Cancer Research Institute (NCRI) Lymphoma Group RAPID trial, patients who were PET negative after 3 cycles of ABVD were randomized to radiotherapy or no further treatment. The German HD16 trial for early-stage patients without risk factors uses up-front randomization, between a standard combined-modality arm and a PET-driven experimental arm, in which patients who are PET negative after 2 cycles of ABVD receive no further treatment.[35] The experimental arms of the European Organisation for Research and Treatment of Cancer (EORTC)/Groupe des Etudes des Lymphomes de l'Adulte (GELA)/Fondazione Italiana Linfomi (FIL) H10 protocol also omitted radiotherapy to early PET-negative patients while escalating to BEACOPPesc followed by radiotherapy in PET-positive patients. This trial tested the noninferiority of a less toxic treatment to good-risk patients, and at the same time attempted treatment intensification for patients regarded as having a high risk of failure based on a positive interim PET/CT. The German HD16 trial is still recruiting patients, but results from the RAPID (Response-Adapted PET trial In early-stage Hodgkin's Disease) trial and the H10 trial were presented at the 2013 annual meeting of the American Society of Hematology.[36,37] The results are

Table 2
Studies of early PET response–adapted therapy in early-stage HL

Study Title	Reference #	Patients	Design	Study Type
GHSG HD16	35	Early-stage HL no risk factors	No radiotherapy in experimental arm if PET-negative after 2 × ABVD	Phase III
EORTC/GELA/FIL H10 (completed)	36	Early-stage HL	Experimental arm: no radiotherapy if PET negative after 2 × ABVD BEACOPPesc + radiotherapy if PET positive after 2 × ABVD	Phase III
UK NCRI RAPID (completed)	37	Early-stage HL	If PET negative after 3 × ABVD, randomization to RT vs no RT	Phase III
CALGB 50604	38	Early-stage HL, nonbulky	Additional ABVD × 2 and no RT if PET negative after 2 × ABVD BEACOPPesc + radiotherapy if PET positive after 2 × ABVD	Phase II
CALGB 50801	39	Early-stage HL, bulky	Additional ABVD × 4 and no RT if PET negative after 2 × ABVD BEACOPPesc + radiotherapy if PET positive after 2 × ABVD	Phase II
ECOG 2410	40	Early-stage HL, bulky	4 × BEACOPPesc + RT if PET positive after 2 × ABVD	Phase II

Abbreviations: CALGB, Cancer and Leukemia Group B; ECOG, Eastern Cooperative Oncology Group; EORTC, European Organisation for Research and Treatment of Cancer; FIL, Fondazione Italiana Linfomi; GELA, Groupe des Etudes des Lymphomes de l'Adulte; GHSG, German Hodgkin Study Group; NCRI, National Cancer Research Institute; RAPID, Response-Adapted PET trial In early-stage Hodgkin's Disease; RT, radiotherapy.

summarized in **Table 3**. The results from the RAPID trial were based on a mature analysis with a median follow-up of 46 months, whereas the H10 results were based on an interim analysis after a median follow-up of 13 months. Apart from this, the results were similar. Early PET-negative patients who, according to randomization, did or did not receive radiotherapy showed differences in PFS rates that were within the predefined margin of noninferiority (7% for RAPID, 10% for H10). Nevertheless, the conclusions from the two studies were the opposite of one another. The RAPID trial is considered a positive trial, because mature results show what is considered noninferiority of the experimental arm. In contrast, the experimental arms for early PET-negative patients in the H10 trial were closed after a futility analysis of the presented interim data rendered it unlikely that noninferiority of the chemotherapy-only treatment could be shown in a mature analysis, compared with the combined-modality standard arms. This analysis used the assumption that the hazard ratio for recurrences in each

Table 3
Preliminary results of H10 and RAPID trials

EORTC/GELA/FIL H10 Trial (Ref.[36])	UK NCRI RAPID Trial (Ref.[37])
1137 patients, median follow-up 13 mo	600 patients, median follow-up 46 mo
Futility analysis based on 33 events	Final analysis based on 36 events
Noninferiority margin 10%	Noninferiority margin 7%
PET2-negative patients without risk factors: • 1-y PFS 94.9% if no radiotherapy • 1-y PFS 100% if INRT	PET3-negative patients: • 3-y PFS 90.7% if no radiotherapy • 3-y PFS 93.8% if IFRT
PET2-negative patients with risk factors: • 1-y PFS 94.7% if no radiotherapy • 1-y PFS 97.3% if INRT	PET3-negative patients: • 3-y OS 99.5% if no radiotherapy • 3-y OS 97.0% if IFRT
Trial closed early because of futility	Trial considered positive

arm is unchanged during the observation period. This assumption is not correct, because most recurrences in HL occur within the first 2 years, and because it is likely that patients not receiving radiotherapy will relapse earlier than those relapsing after combined-modality treatment.

Meanwhile, 2 ongoing North American phase II trials are investigating FDG-PET after 2 cycles of ABVD for selection of patients who are eligible for treatment with chemotherapy alone. The Cancer and Leukemia Group B (CALGB) 50604 and 50801 trials assess strategies that are similar to the experimental arms of the EORTC/GELA/IIL H10 trial. In these trials, patients PET-negative after 2 cycles of ABVD are treated with ABVD alone (4 and 6 cycles for patients without and with bulky disease, respectively), whereas patients who are PET positive after 2 cycles of ABVD proceed to 2 cycles of BEACOPPesc followed by 30-Gy IFRT.[38,39] In the ECOG 2410 phase II trial for early-stage patients with bulky disease, 2 cycles of ABVD are followed by FDG-PET, which determines whether the patients continue with another 4 cycles of ABVD or proceed to 4 cycles of BEACOPPesc. In this trial, all patients are given 30-Gy INRT after completion of chemotherapy.[40]

The numerous observational studies of interim FDG-PET show that an early negative FDG-PET identifies a group of patients in whom more than 90% will achieve long-term PFS even without radiotherapy. Early PET-negative patients with early-stage disease and without bulk/risk factors are likely to be treated safely without radiotherapy. In contrast, the presented data from the H10 trial and the RAPID trial show that the omission of radiotherapy will probably result in a slightly reduced local tumor control and PFS, even in patients without risk factors. A certain PFS inferiority of the PET response–adapted strategy may be acceptable, particularly if, as could be expected, the PFS difference is caused by an increased number of patients with local, early relapses that may be treated effectively with radiotherapy.

Overall, it is still uncertain whether PET/CT can select patients with early-stage HL who may be safely treated without radiotherapy, and the German HD16 trial results are highly anticipated. Longer follow-up and results from more of the ongoing trials are awaited. Of particular interest are the following questions:

- What are the differences in PFS and OS between PET response–adapted therapy and combined-modality therapy after 3 to 5 years, by which point most local recurrences have occurred?
- How many of the patients who relapse early (<1 year) after chemotherapy alone can be cured by radiotherapy (ie, without the need for high-dose chemotherapy)?

- In contrast, how many more patients treated initially with chemotherapy alone will eventually need high-dose salvage therapy to achieve cure?

Until these questions are answered, a PET response–adapted treatment approach outside clinical trials should be discouraged.

PET RESPONSE–ADAPTED HL THERAPY: ADVANCED-STAGE DISEASE

Around 65% to 70% of patients with advanced-stage HL are cured with 6 to 8 cycles of ABVD with or without consolidation radiotherapy, which is first-line therapy in most centers. BEACOPPesc cures around 85% of patients if given up-front, but serious concerns regarding acute toxicity and second myeloid neoplasias are the reason why many centers in Europe and North America are reluctant to use this regimen as standard therapy.[41–43] Like in early-stage disease, the pretreatment prognostic tools, notably the IPS, does not accurately predict which patients need more intensive therapy. As noted previously, a negative early interim FDG-PET is a strong predictor of a favorable outcome with standard therapy. Studies have consistently shown long-term PFS rates of approximately 95% in early PET-negative patients with advanced-stage HL treated with ABVD.[17–20] Based on these findings, several trials investigating PET response–adapted therapy for patients with advanced-stage HL are ongoing or recently completed (**Table 4**). The general aim of these trials is to deescalate therapy to those patients with a good early PET response, to escalate therapy to those patients who do not respond well, or to do both.

Completed Trials

The nonrandomized Italian GITIL (Gruppo Italiano Terapie Innovative nei Linfomi) HD0607 trial used early treatment intensification with BEACOPPesc in patients who were still PET positive after 2 cycles of ABVD, resulting in 2-year OS of 98% for the cohort, and 92% and 65% failure-free survival for early PET-negative and PET-positive patients, respectively.[44] Other similar trial is the UK-Nordic RATHL trial, which completed recruitment recently. In the RATHL trial, early PET-positive patients proceeded to BEACOPP therapy, whereas early PET-negative patients were randomized to either continued ABVD or to Adriamycin, vinblastine, and dacarbazine (ie, omission of bleomycin for the last 4 therapy cycles). No mature outcome data from the RATHL study have been published, but a recent presentation showed that, among the early PET-positive patients, 74% reached a negative postchemotherapy FDG-PET after having been shifted to BEACOPP therapy.[45] The Israeli group have published their long-term experience with PET response–tailored BEACOPP-based therapy for advanced HL, showing excellent cure rates in patients treated with the less intensive BEACOPP-baseline in cases of a negative FDG-PET after the first 2 cycles of either BEACOPPesc or BEACOPPbaseline (depending on pretreatment IPS).[46] Also, preliminary results from the Italian HD0801 phase II trial have been reported. In this trial, patients with advanced-stage HL were offered high-dose chemotherapy with autologous stem cell support (HD+ASCT) in cases of a positive FDG-PET after 2 cycles of ABVD. The available data are immature, so it is currently not possible to judge whether this intensive escalation of therapy can be justified in early PET-positive patients.[47]

Ongoing Trials

Several trials are ongoing. The randomized German GHSG HD18 trial tests abbreviation of BEACOPPesc therapy based on PET results after 2 therapy cycles.[48] The French AHL 2011 trial is also a BEACOPPesc-based randomized trial with treatment modifications based on PET after both 2 and 4 cycles.[49] The recently opened EORTC/PLRG H11

Table 4
Studies of early PET response–adapted therapy in advanced-stage HL

Study Title	Reference #	Patients	Design	Study Type
GITIL HD0607 (completed)	44	Stage IIB–IV + stage IIA with RF	Intensification to BEACOPPesc if PET positive after 2 × ABVD	Phase II
RATHL (completed)	45	Stage IIB–IV	Intensification to BEACOPP if PET positive after 2 × ABVD randomization between ABVD and AVD if PET negative	Phase III
Israel/Rambam (completed)	46	Early stage + RF/bulk or advanced stage	PET after 2 × BEACOPPbaseline or BEACOPPesc: proceed to 4 × BEACOPPesc if PET positive or 4 × BEACOPPbaseline if PET negative	Phase II
IIL HD0801 (completed)	47	Stage IIB–IV	Salvage regimen if PET positive after 2 × ABVD. Randomization between radiotherapy and no further treatment after completion of 6 × ABVD if PET negative after 2 × ABVD	Phase III
GHSG HD18	48	Early-stage HL, bulky	4 vs 6 × BEACOPPesc in experimental arm if PET negative after 2 cycles. Standard arm: 6 × BEACOPPesc	Phase III
LYSA AHL2011	49	Early-stage HL, bulky	De-escalation from BEACOPPesc to ABVD in experimental arm in case of a negative PET after 2 and 4 cycles. Standard arm: 6 × BEACOPPesc	Phase III
EORTC/PLRG H11	50	Stage III–IV	Experimental arm: intensification to BEACOPPesc if PET positive after 1 × ABVD. Standard arm: 6 × BEACOPPesc	Phase III
SWOG S0816	51	Stage III–IV	Intensification to BEACOPPesc if PET positive after 2 × ABVD	Phase II

Abbreviation: AVD, adriamycin, vinblastine, and dacarbazine.

trial compares BEACOPPesc (standard arm) against an experimental arm in which PET/CT after 1 cycle of ABVD determines whether patients continue with ABVD or BEACOP-Pesc.[50] In addition, the ongoing Southwestern Oncology Group (SWOG) S0816 study is a phase II trial with a design similar to that of the Italian GITIL HD0607 trial.[51]

THE IMPORTANCE OF INTERPRETATION CRITERIA

The understanding of the published observational studies of interim FDG-PET and of some of the published PET response–adapted HL therapy studies is complicated by these studies having used a wide range of different criteria for interim PET interpretation. These criteria have in general been well defined and generally not validated. FDG-PET results are not easily divided into positive and negative groups, because FDG uptake represents a continuum and not a dichotomous phenomenon. The threshold between positive and negative (including the handling of complicated, equivocal results) has a great impact on the results of PET-driven trials. In addition, for trial results to be comparable, applicable, and reproducible outside of clinical trials, the interpretation criteria must not only offer an accurate prediction of outcome but also must be simple and reproducible. For this reason, the community of nuclear medicine experts and lymphoma therapists has met regularly in recent years and gathered data in order to agree on such criteria.[24,52,53] There is now a general agreement to use the Deauville criteria, which are a 5-point scale reflecting FDG uptake in the initially involved lymphoma tissues (**Box 1**). The threshold between a negative and a positive scan can be set between scores 2 and 3, or between scores 3 and 4, depending on whether a high negative predictive value is desirable (in de-escalation strategies) or whether a high positive predictive value is preferred (in escalation strategies). The Deauville criteria have replaced the posttreatment reading criteria developed by Juweid and colleagues[54] for the 2007 revision of the international lymphoma response criteria,[55] because several studies have shown higher accuracy and superior interobserver agreement when using the 5-point scale.[23,56] The use of semiquantitative measurements of FDG uptake has been proposed in order to further reduce interobserver variation, but no studies have so far shown a clear advantage compared with visual assessment. Equally important as standardized interpretation criteria is the adherence to international guidelines for image acquisition and quality control; however, these are outside the scope of this article.[57]

POSTCHEMOTHERAPY FDG-PET/CT FOR SELECTION OF PATIENTS FOR CONSOLIDATION RADIOTHERAPY

In advanced disease, radiotherapy is used less frequently and usually only for residual disease. In this situation, FDG-PET may help in discriminating between a residual

---

Box 1
Deauville criteria for interpretation of PET in lymphoma

1. No pathologic FDG uptake

2. Uptake less than or equal to mediastinum

3. Uptake greater than mediastinum but less than or equal to liver

4. Uptake moderately higher than liver

5. Uptake markedly higher than liver and/or new lesions

X. New areas of uptake unlikely to be related to lymphoma.

mass with viable lymphoma cells and a residual mass consisting only of fibrotic tissue. A large number of studies have shown a high negative predictive value of FDG-PET/CT after completion of therapy for HL, as documented in a recent meta-analysis.[58] However, because FDG-PET cannot detect microscopic disease, it has not been clear whether a PET-negative residual mass requires radiotherapy. The mature results of the German HD15 trial shed light on this for patients treated with BEACOPP regimens. In this study, consolidation radiotherapy was given only to patients with a PET-positive residual mass of more than 2.5 cm. The remaining patients who did not receive radiotherapy had a relapse-free survival of 94% after 1 year, indicating that radiotherapy can safely be omitted in patients with advanced-stage HL who are PET-negative after the end of BEACOPPesc. The situation is less clear for ABVD-treated patients. Retrospective data from the British Columbia Cancer Agency were presented at the Annual Meeting of the American Society of Clinical Oncology in 2011. This retrospective study reported a 5-year experience in which patients with residual masses larger than 2 cm after chemotherapy underwent FDG-PET/CT (n = 163). Only posttreatment PET-positive patients received radiotherapy. Of the patients with a negative PET/CT (n = 130, 80%), the 3-year PFS was 89% with a median follow-up of 34 months, as opposed to the PET-positive patients who had a 3-year PFS of 55% despite receiving radiotherapy.[59] These results strongly support the omission of radiotherapy to patients with advanced-stage HL who achieve a PET-negative remission after 6 cycles of chemotherapy.

The ongoing GHSG HD17 trial investigates omission of radiotherapy in early-stage unfavorable disease (including patients with bulky disease and other risk factors). In this trial, patients who are PET negative after 2 cycles of BEACOPPesc plus 2 cycles of ABVD are randomized to either 30-Gy IFRT (standard treatment) or no further treatment. No results from this large ongoing trial have been reported.[60]

PET/CT BEFORE HIGH-DOSE SALVAGE THERAPY IN RELAPSED HL

For relapsed patients or patients with primary refractory HL undergoing HD+ASCT, the duration of remission before relapse and the response to induction therapy are the most important prognostic factors that predict final outcome. Several studies have shown that FDG-PET performed after induction therapy and before HD+ASCT can predict which patients with HL will achieve long-term remission.[61–63] These studies all report a poor long-term PFS (after 2–5 years) in patients who are PET positive after induction chemotherapy (31%–41%), compared with a PFS of 73% to 82% in patients who reach a PET-negative remission before HD+ASCT. However, these studies also report a higher false-positive rate than with PET/CT performed early during first-line therapy. The role of PET/CT in this setting is still unclear, but there is a need for clinical trials in order to improve the outcomes for patients who are still PET positive after induction salvage chemotherapy. Encouraging results were published recently by Moscowitz and colleagues,[64] who showed that a PET-guided approach may help these patients. In this study, patients who were still PET positive after the standard induction regimen (ifosfamide, carboplatin, and etoposide [ICE]) did not proceed to HD+ASCT but instead to a non–cross-resistant regimen consisting of 4 biweekly doses of gemcitabine, vinorelbine, and liposomal doxorubicin (GVD) before HD+ASCT. Those patients who converted to being PET negative after GVD and before HD+ASCT had similar outcomes to those who were PET negative after ICE and went on with the initially planned HD+ASCT. In a currently recruiting trial, the same institution will offer brentuximab vedotin (BV) as induction therapy to patients with HL in first relapse. FDG-PET after 2 cycles of BV determines whether the patients proceed directly to HD+ASCT or shift to the ICE regimen (in cases of a positive FDG-PET).[65]

PET/CT IN PATIENTS WHO RELAPSED AFTER SECOND-LINE THERAPY

Little is known about PET/CT in patients who relapse after, or who are ineligible for, HD+ASCT. The remission status determined by PET/CT before allogeneic stem cell transplantation with reduced-intensity conditioning seems to be highly predictive of outcome.[66] Two studies indicate that, after allogeneic stem cell transplantation, PET/CT may have a role in guiding the use of donor lymphocyte infusions.[67,68] The remission status determined by FDG-PET/CT seems to strongly predict PFS in patients with relapsed/refractory HL treated with BV.[69]

SUMMARY

FDG-PET/CT is the most important imaging modality in the management of HL and the most accurate tool for staging, treatment monitoring, and response evaluation. This verdict is based on an extensive number of observational studies performed over the last 15 years. Although FDG-PET/CT seems to exceed any other existing tools in terms of diagnostic and prognostic properties, its clinical value to patients depends on the way clinicians use it. There is a general agreement that it is desirable to have access to the most accurate determination of disease extent at the time of diagnosis, and also to have access to the most prognostic assessment of final treatment response. For those reasons, PET/CT has been accepted as standard of care at staging and final response assessment of HL, and consequently is incorporated into the current guidelines.

The situation is less clear during therapy. The therapeutic dilemma in HL is that both early-stage and advanced-stage patients have high cure rates but have serious long-term treatment-related morbidity and mortality. Because most patients are subject to some overtreatment, a minority of patients does not achieve a lasting remission and might benefit from more intensive first-line therapy. FDG-PET is the best tool at hand for response-adapted therapy for HL designed to stratify treatment according to early assessment of treatment sensitivity.

A large number of recently completed and ongoing trials have investigated such early PET response–adapted therapy. Until mature results are available, the use of PET response–adapted therapy should not be encouraged outside clinical trials.

In summary:
- Is interim FDG-PET a safe predictor of final response and outcome? Yes.
- Is FDG-PET a safe predictor for a change of therapy? Perhaps.

REFERENCES

1. Evens AM, Hutchings M, Diehl V. Treatment of Hodgkin lymphoma: the past, present, and future. Nat Clin Pract Oncol 2008;5:543–56.
2. Hancock SL, Hoppe RT. Long-term complications of treatment and causes of mortality after Hodgkin's disease. Semin Radiat Oncol 1996;6:225–42.
3. Hoppe RT. Hodgkin's disease: complications of therapy and excess mortality. Ann Oncol 1997;8(Suppl 1):115–8.
4. Engert A, Plutschow A, Eich HT, et al. Reduced treatment intensity in patients with early-stage Hodgkin's lymphoma. N Engl J Med 2010;363:640–52.
5. Eich HT, Diehl V, Gorgen H, et al. Intensified chemotherapy and dose-reduced involved-field radiotherapy in patients with early unfavorable Hodgkin's

lymphoma: final analysis of the German Hodgkin Study Group HD11 Trial. J Clin Oncol 2010;28:4199–206.

6. Bonadonna G, Viviani S, Bonfante V, et al. Survival in Hodgkin's disease patients: report of 25 years of experience at the Milan Cancer Institute. Eur J Cancer 2005;41:998–1006.

7. Engert A, Haverkamp H, Kobe C, et al. Reduced-intensity chemotherapy and PET-guided radiotherapy in patients with advanced stage Hodgkin's lymphoma (HD15 trial): a randomised, open-label, phase 3 non-inferiority trial. Lancet 2012;379(9828):1791–9.

8. Hoppe RT, Advani RH, Ai WZ, et al. Hodgkin lymphoma. J Natl Compr Canc Netw 2011;9:1020–58.

9. Engert A, Eichenauer DA, Dreyling M. Hodgkin's lymphoma: ESMO clinical practice guidelines for diagnosis, treatment and follow-up. Ann Oncol 2010; 21(Suppl 5):v168–71.

10. Specht L, Yahalom J, Illidge T, et al. Modern radiation therapy for Hodgkin lymphoma: field and dose guidelines from the International Lymphoma Radiation Oncology Group (ILROG). Int J Radiat Oncol Biol Phys 2013. [Epub ahead of print].

11. Hutchings M. How does PET/CT help in selecting therapy for patients with Hodgkin lymphoma? Hematology Am Soc Hematol Educ Program 2012;2012:322–7.

12. Hutchings M, Barrington SF. PET/CT for therapy response assessment in lymphoma. J Nucl Med 2009;50(Suppl 1):21S–30S.

13. Rankin SC. Assessment of response to therapy using conventional imaging. Eur J Nucl Med Mol Imaging 2003;30(Suppl 1):S56–64.

14. Canellos GP. Residual mass in lymphoma may not be residual disease. J Clin Oncol 1988;6:931–3.

15. Zinzani PL, Tani M, Fanti S, et al. Early positron emission tomography (PET) restaging: a predictive final response in Hodgkin's disease patients. Ann Oncol 2006;17:1296–300.

16. Hutchings M, Mikhaeel NG, Fields PA, et al. Prognostic value of interim FDG-PET after two or three cycles of chemotherapy in Hodgkin lymphoma. Ann Oncol 2005;16:1160–8.

17. Hutchings M, Loft A, Hansen M, et al. FDG-PET after two cycles of chemotherapy predicts treatment failure and progression-free survival in Hodgkin lymphoma. Blood 2006;107:52–9.

18. Gallamini A, Rigacci L, Merli F, et al. The predictive value of positron emission tomography scanning performed after two courses of standard therapy on treatment outcome in advanced stage Hodgkin's disease. Haematologica 2006;91: 475–81.

19. Gallamini A, Hutchings M, Rigacci L, et al. Early interim 2-[18F]fluoro-2-deoxy-D-glucose positron emission tomography is prognostically superior to international prognostic score in advanced-stage Hodgkin's lymphoma: a report from a joint Italian-Danish study. J Clin Oncol 2007;25:3746–52.

20. Cerci JJ, Pracchia LF, Linardi CC, et al. 18F-FDG PET after 2 cycles of ABVD predicts event-free survival in early and advanced Hodgkin lymphoma. J Nucl Med 2010;51:1337–43.

21. Kostakoglu L, Goldsmith SJ, Leonard JP, et al. FDG-PET after 1 cycle of therapy predicts outcome in diffuse large cell lymphoma and classic Hodgkin disease. Cancer 2006;107:2678–87.

22. Zinzani P, Rigacci L, Stefoni V, et al. Early interim 18F-FDG PET in Hodgkin's lymphoma: evaluation on 304 patients. Eur J Nucl Med Mol Imaging 2012;39:4–12.

23. Biggi A, Gallamini A, Chauvie S, et al. International validation study for interim PET in ABVD-treated, advanced-stage Hodgkin lymphoma: interpretation criteria and concordance rate among reviewers. J Nucl Med 2013;54: 683–90.
24. Meignan M, Gallamini A, Meignan M, et al. Report on the first international workshop on interim-PET scan in lymphoma. Leuk Lymphoma 2009;50: 1257–60.
25. Hutchings M, Kostakoglu L, Zaucha JM, et al. Early determination of treatment sensitivity in Hodgkin lymphoma: FDG-PET/CT has a higher negative predictive value after one cycle of therapy than after two cycles of chemotherapy. Ann Oncol 2011;22:iv138–9.
26. Markova J, Kahraman D, Kobe C, et al. Role of [18F]-fluoro-2-deoxy-D-glucose positron emission tomography in early and late therapy assessment of patients with advanced Hodgkin lymphoma treated with bleomycin, etoposide, Adriamycin, cyclophosphamide, vincristine, procarbazine and prednisone. Leuk Lymphoma 2012;53:64–70.
27. Filippi AR, Botticella A, Bello B, et al. Interim positron emission tomography and clinical outcome in patients with early stage Hodgkin lymphoma treated with combined modality therapy. Leuk Lymphoma 2012;54:1183–7.
28. Kostakoglu L, Schoder H, Johnson JL, et al. Interim [18F]fluorodeoxyglucose positron emission tomography imaging in stage I-II non-bulky Hodgkin lymphoma: would using combined positron emission tomography and computed tomography criteria better predict response than each test alone? Leuk Lymphoma 2012;53:2143–50.
29. Aleman BM, van den Belt-Dusebout AW, Klokman WJ, et al. Long-term cause-specific mortality of patients treated for Hodgkin's disease. J Clin Oncol 2003; 21:3431–9.
30. Ferme C, Eghbali H, Meerwaldt JH, et al. Chemotherapy plus involved-field radiation in early-stage Hodgkin's disease. N Engl J Med 2007;357: 1916–27.
31. Noordijk EM, Carde P, Dupouy NL, et al. Combined-modality therapy for clinical stage I or II Hodgkin's lymphoma: long-term results of the European Organisation for Research and Treatment of Cancer H7 randomized controlled trials. J Clin Oncol 2006;24:3128–35.
32. Engert A, Schiller P, Josting A, et al. Involved-field radiotherapy is equally effective and less toxic compared with extended-field radiotherapy after four cycles of chemotherapy in patients with early-stage unfavorable Hodgkin's lymphoma: results of the HD8 trial of the German Hodgkin's Lymphoma Study Group. J Clin Oncol 2003;21:3601–8.
33. Meyer RM, Gospodarowicz MK, Connors JM, et al. ABVD alone versus radiation-based therapy in limited-stage Hodgkin's lymphoma. N Engl J Med 2011;366:399–408.
34. von Tresckow B, Plütschow A, Fuchs M, et al. Dose-intensification in early unfavorable Hodgkin's lymphoma: final analysis of the German Hodgkin Study Group HD14 Trial. J Clin Oncol 2012;30:907–13.
35. HD16 for early stage Hodgkin lymphoma. 2008. Available at: http://www.clinicaltrials.gov/ct2/show/NCT00736320.
36. Andre MP, Reman O, Federico M, et al. Interim analysis of the randomized EORTC/LYSA/FIL Intergroup H10 trial on early pet-scan driven treatment adaptation in stage I/II Hodgkin lymphoma. ASH Annual Meeting Abstracts 2012;120: 549.

37. Radford J, O'Doherty M, Barrington S, et al. Results of the 2nd planned interim analysis of the RAPID Trial (involved field radiotherapy versus no further treatment) in patients with clinical stages 1A and 2A Hodgkin lymphoma and a 'negative' FDG-PET scan after 3 cycles ABVD. ASH Annual Meeting Abstracts 2008;112:369.

38. Chemotherapy Based on Positron Emission Tomography Scan in Treating Patients With Stage I or Stage II Hodgkin Lymphoma. 2013. Available at: http://clinicaltrials.gov/ct2/show/NCT01132807.

39. Response-Based Therapy Assessed By PET Scan in Treating Patients With Bulky Stage I and Stage II Classical Hodgkin Lymphoma. 2013. Available at: http://clinicaltrials.gov/ct2/show/NCT01118026.

40. Chemotherapy Based on PET Scan in Treating Patients With Stage I or Stage II Hodgkin Lymphoma. 2013. Available at: http://clinicaltrials.gov/ct2/show/NCT01390584.

41. Engert A, Diehl V, Franklin J, et al. Escalated-dose BEACOPP in the treatment of patients with advanced-stage Hodgkin's lymphoma: 10 years of follow-up of the GHSG HD9 study. J Clin Oncol 2009;27:4548–54.

42. Federico M, Luminari S, Iannitto E, et al. ABVD compared with BEACOPP compared with CEC for the initial treatment of patients with advanced Hodgkin's lymphoma: results from the HD2000 Gruppo Italiano per lo Studio dei Linfomi Trial. J Clin Oncol 2009;27:805–11.

43. Viviani S, Zinzani PL, Rambaldi A, et al. ABVD versus BEACOPP for Hodgkin's lymphoma when high-dose salvage is planned. N Engl J Med 2011;365:203–12.

44. Gallamini A, Patti C, Viviani S, et al. Early chemotherapy intensification with BEACOPP in advanced-stage Hodgkin lymphoma patients with a interim-PET positive after two ABVD courses. Br J Haematol 2011;152:551–60.

45. Johnson P, Federico M, Fossa A, et al. Responses and chemotherapy dose adjustment determined by PET-CT imaging: first results from the international Response Adapted Therapy in Advanced Hodgkin Lymphoma (RATHL) study [abstract]. Hematol Oncol 2013;31:138.

46. Dann EJ, Blumenfeld Z, Bar-Shalom R, et al. A 10-year experience with treatment of high and standard risk Hodgkin disease: six cycles of tailored BEACOPP, with interim scintigraphy, are effective and female fertility is preserved. Am J Hematol 2012;87:32–6.

47. Zinzani PL, Bonfichi M, Rossi G, et al. Interim results of IIL-HD0801 study on early salvage with high-dose chemotherapy and stem cell transplantation in advanced Hodgkin's lymphoma patients with positive positron emission tomography after two courses of chemotherapy [abstract]. Hematol Oncol 2013;31:102.

48. HD18 for advanced stages in Hodgkins lymphoma. 2008. Available at: http://www.clinicaltrials.gov/ct2/show/NCT00515554.

49. Study of a treatment driven by early PET response to a treatment not monitored by early PET in patients with AA stage 3-4 or 2B HL (AHL 2011). 2013. Available at: http://clinicaltrials.gov/ct2/show/NCT01358747.

50. Very early FDG-PET/CT-response adapted therapy for advanced Hodgkin lymphoma (H11). 2013. Available at: http://www.clinicaltrials.gov/ct2/show/NCT01652261.

51. Fludeoxyglucose F 18-PET/CT imaging and combination chemotherapy with or without additional chemotherapy and G-CSF in treating patients with stage III or stage IV Hodgkin lymphoma. 2013. Available at: http://clinicaltrials.gov/ct2/show/NCT00822120.

52. Meignan M, Gallamini A, Haioun C, et al. Report on the Second International Workshop on Interim Positron Emission Tomography in Lymphoma held in Menton, France, 8–9 April 2010. Leuk Lymphoma 2010;51:2171–80.
53. Meignan M, Barrington SF, Itti E, et al. Report on the 4th International workshop on Positron Emission Tomography in Lymphoma held in Menton, France, 3–5 October 2012. Leuk Lymphoma 2013. [E-pub ahead of print].
54. Juweid ME, Stroobants S, Hoekstra OS, et al. Use of positron emission tomography for response assessment of lymphoma: consensus of the Imaging Subcommittee of International Harmonization Project in Lymphoma. J Clin Oncol 2007;25:571–8.
55. Cheson BD, Pfistner B, Juweid ME, et al. Revised response criteria for malignant lymphoma. J Clin Oncol 2007;25:579–86.
56. Barrington SF, Qian W, Somer EJ, et al. Concordance between four European centres of PET reporting criteria designed for use in multicentre trials in Hodgkin lymphoma. Eur J Nucl Med Mol Imaging 2010;37:1824–33.
57. Boellaard R, O'Doherty M, Weber W, et al. FDG PET and PET/CT: EANM procedure guidelines for tumour PET imaging: version 1.0. Eur J Nucl Med Mol Imaging 2010;37:181–200.
58. Terasawa T, Nihashi T, Hotta T, et al. 18F-FDG PET for posttherapy assessment of Hodgkin's disease and aggressive non-Hodgkin's lymphoma: a systematic review. J Nucl Med 2008;49:13–21.
59. Savage KJ, Connors JM, Klasa RJ, et al. The use of FDG-PET to guide consolidative radiotherapy in patients with advanced-stage Hodgkin lymphoma with residual abnormalities on CT scan following ABVD chemotherapy. J Clin Oncol 2011;29 [abstract].
60. HD17 for intermediate stage Hodgkin lymphoma. 2013. Available at: http://clinicaltrials.gov/ct2/show/NCT01356680.
61. Mocikova H, Pytlik R, Markova J, et al. Pre-transplant positron emission tomography in relapsed Hodgkin lymphoma patients. Leuk Lymphoma 2011;52(9):1668–74.
62. Smeltzer JP, Cashen AF, Zhang Q, et al. Prognostic significance of FDG-PET in relapsed or refractory classical Hodgkin lymphoma treated with standard salvage chemotherapy and autologous stem cell transplantation. Biol Blood Marrow Transplant 2011;17:1646–52.
63. Moskowitz AJ, Yahalom J, Kewalramani T, et al. Pretransplantation functional imaging predicts outcome following autologous stem cell transplantation for relapsed and refractory Hodgkin lymphoma. Blood 2010;116:4934–7.
64. Moskowitz CH, Matasar MJ, Zelenetz AD, et al. Normalization of pre-ASCT, FDG-PET imaging with second-line, non-cross-resistant, chemotherapy programs improves event-free survival in patients with Hodgkin lymphoma. Blood 2012;119:1665–70.
65. Brentuximab Vedotin (SGN-35) in transplant eligible patients with relapsed or refractory Hodgkin lymphoma. 2013. Available at: http://clinicaltrials.gov/ct2/show/NCT01508312.
66. Dodero A, Crocchiolo R, Patriarca F, et al. Pretransplantation [18-F] fluorodeoxyglucose positron emission tomography scan predicts outcome in patients with recurrent Hodgkin lymphoma or aggressive non-Hodgkin lymphoma undergoing reduced-intensity conditioning followed by allogeneic stem cell transplantation. Cancer 2010;116:5001–11.
67. Lambert JR, Bomanji JB, Peggs KS, et al. Prognostic role of PET scanning before and after reduced-intensity allogeneic stem cell transplantation for lymphoma. Blood 2010;115:2763–8.

68. Hart DP, Avivi I, Thomson KJ, et al. Use of 18F-FDG positron emission tomography following allogeneic transplantation to guide adoptive immunotherapy with donor lymphocyte infusions. Br J Haematol 2005;128:824–9.
69. Younes A, Gopal AK, Smith SE, et al. Results of a pivotal phase II study of brentuximab vedotin for patients with relapsed or refractory Hodgkin's lymphoma. J Clin Oncol 2012;30:2183–9.

Customized Targeted Therapy in Hodgkin Lymphoma: Hype or Hope?

Catherine Diefenbach, MD[a], Ranjana Advani, MD[b],*

KEYWORDS

- Hodgkin lymphoma • Relapsed disease • Targeted therapies • Brentuximab vedotin

KEY POINTS

- Patients with Hodgkin lymphoma (HL) with primary refractory disease or relapse after transplant have poor outcomes and represent an unmet need.
- Therapies derived from an understanding of HL biology can be broadly classified as targeting the Hodgkin Reed Sternberg cell-surface receptors, tumor microenvironment, cell-mediated immunity, and intracellular signaling pathways.
- Brentuximab vedotin, an antibody-drug conjugate targeting CD30 now approved by the Food and Drug Administration, offers substantial hope for improving outcomes in the treatment of HL.
- Other therapies in development need longer follow-up to realize their potential.

Objectives
1. Review recent advances in HL biology
2. Review development of novel targeted therapies in the context of HL biology
3. Review results of clinical trials with targeted therapies

INTRODUCTION

Classic Hodgkin lymphoma (HL) represents approximately 10% of all lymphomas diagnosed annually in the developing world. In 2013, approximately 9000 cases of HL were diagnosed in the United States.[1] With a median age of 38 years, and at least 40% of patients younger than 35 years at the time of diagnosis, it is the most common

Disclosures of Potential Conflicts of Interest: Catherine Diefenbach: Seattle Genetics, consulting and speakers bureau. Ranjana Advani: Seattle Genetics, research funding and advisory board; Genentech, advisory board and research funding; Millennium: The Takeda Oncology Company, research and advisory board.
Catherine Diefenbach is supported in part by the NYU Clinical and Translational Science Institute (CTSI) NIH/NCATS UL1 TR00038.
[a] Department of Medicine, New York University School of Medicine/New York University Cancer Center, 240 East 38th Street, New York, NY 10016, USA; [b] Medicine/Oncology, Stanford Cancer Center, Stanford University Medical Center, 875 Blake Wilbur Drive, Stanford, CA 94305, USA
* Corresponding author.
E-mail address: radvani@stanford.edu

lymphoma affecting young patients.[2] Over the past 30 years, valuable lessons learned about the late effects of therapy, specifically cardiovascular and second cancer risk, have led to treatment modifications of radiation dose and field size as well as alkylator exposure, which have led to significant risk reduction of competing causes of death.[3,4,5] As a result of these advances, more than 75% of patients are cured with contemporary frontline therapy.[6,7]

For patients who relapse after attaining an initial complete remission (CR) or have primary refractory disease, the standard treatment approach is salvage chemotherapy followed by autologous stem cell transplant (ASCT), with an approximately 50% cure rate.[8] Several studies show that achieving a CR before ASCT is one of the most important factors in determining a long-term outcome after ASCT.[9,10] Other pretransplant prognostic factors include duration of initial remission, extent of disease at relapse, and constitutional symptoms.[11,12,13,14] In an international collaborative effort from 5 countries, data on 756 patients with relapsed HL with a minimum of 1-year follow-up after the transplant were pooled.[15] The overall median postprogression survival (PPS) for patients relapsing after ASCT was 1.3 years. Seventy-one percent of relapses occurred within 1 year after ASCT and were roughly equally distributed in the following periods: less than 3 months (22%), more than 3 and less than 6 months (22%), and more than 6 and less than 12 months (27%). The median PPS for these periods were 0.55, 1.6, 1.68, and 2.26 years for the time to relapse after ASCT, respectively ($P<.0001$).[15] Allogeneic stem cell transplantation (alloSCT) can induce durable remissions in some of these patients; however, its utility is limited by the challenges of finding an available stem cell donor, and achieving adequate disease control before transplantation.[16] Therefore novel treatments to increase the CR rate pre SCT, or significantly prolong remission duration post SCT, have been sought.

The recent approval in 2011 of brentuximab vedotin, an antibody-drug conjugate (ADC) targeting CD30, has been the first major advance in the management of HL after several decades and offers considerable hope to patients with refractory disease or relapse after stem cell transplant.[17] Better understanding of the biology of HL has led to the exploration of several other potential targets as therapeutic options. This review provides an overview of HL tumor biology in the context of the development of novel targeted therapies. The authors discuss 4 broad categories of targeted therapies either approved or under investigation: (1) therapies targeting Hodgkin Reed Sternberg (HRS) cell-surface receptors, (2) therapies targeting reactive immune cells in the tumor microenvironment, (3) adoptive immunotherapy, and (4) therapies targeting signaling and intracellular survival pathways (**Tables 1** and **2**). Although some of the agents discussed later are highly active as single agents, many others demonstrate modest single-agent activity. Moving forward, the challenge will be how to develop rational combinations of these novel agents within the context of current paradigms of care to achieve enhanced efficacy with minimal toxicity.

EMERGING TARGETS IN THE BIOLOGY OF HL

Classical HL is a B-cell lymphoid neoplasm, characterized by HRS cells. The malignant HRS cells represent only a small fraction (0.1%–1.0%) of the total cellular population and exist within an inflammatory microenvironment that supports tumor growth and suppresses immune surveillance.[18,19,20,21,22] HRS cells grow poorly both in vitro and in vivo murine models without microenvironment support, underscoring its role in HL growth and survival.[19,23] The crosstalk between the HRS cells, the peritumoral cells in the tumor microenvironment, and secreted cytokines propagates HRS cell growth, proliferation, and evasion of immune regulation.

HRS cells express many surface receptors, including CD15, CD30, CD40, CD80, and CD25 (the alpha chain of the interleukin 2 [IL-2] receptor).[24] Additionally, the upregulation of the programed death ligand-1 (PDL-1) on HRS cells induces anergy in peritumoral T cells expressing the receptor programmed death-1 (PD-1). High expression of PD-1 by peritumoral lymphocytes has been reported to be an independent predictor of inferior overall survival (OS).[25,26] Galectin-1 (gal-1) expression inhibits infiltration of CD8+ effector cells, expression of tumor necrosis factor (TNF)-related apoptosis-inducing ligand (TRAIL), and Fas ligand-induced apoptosis of cytotoxic T lymphocytes (CTLs).[27,28] HRS cells further shape their microenvironment by secreting immunosuppressive cytokines and chemokines, such as the chemokine thymus and activation-regulated chemokine/CCL17 (TARC), chemokine ligand 5 (CCL5), and chemokine ligand 22 (CCL22). These, in turn, attract T helper 2 (Th2) and regulatory T (Treg) cells to the tumor microenvironment as well as IL-7, which then induces differentiation of naïve CD4+ T cells toward FoxP3+ Treg cells.[29,30,31] In fact, high serum levels of the chemokine TARC at diagnosis have been associated with an inferior clinical outcome.[32] Tumor-associated macrophages (TAM) induce signal transducer and activator of transcription (STAT) mediated suppression of T-cell surveillance and cell-directed cytotoxicity. Increased numbers of CD68 and CD163 expressing TAMs are also associated with inferior survival in patients with newly diagnosed HL treated with standard therapy as well as in patients following ASCT.[33] Cumulatively, the tumor microenvironment induces T-cell exhaustion and deficient antitumor immunity, which plays a key role in propagating a permissive milieu for HL growth. Although many of the dots of this complex network have been connected, it is still unclear how they all fit together or what is the logical road map for treating relapsed and refractory HL. At a conceptual level, targeted therapies can be broadly classified as targeting (1) HRS cell-surface receptors, (2) the tumor microenvironment, (3) cell-mediated immunity (adoptive immunotherapy), and (4) signaling pathways. **Fig. 1** displays selected novel agents in the context of their targets.

TARGETING MOLECULES EXPRESSED ON HRS CELL SURFACE

Receptors highly expressed on the HRS cell surface, with low to absent expression on normal tissues, are optimal for targeted therapy. Trials evaluating these targets are summarized in **Tables 1** and **2**.

Targeting CD30

CD30 is highly expressed on HRS cells, and nearly absent on normal tissue, making it an optimal target of directed therapy. It is a 120-KDa type I transmembrane glycoprotein belonging to the TNF superfamily and induces signaling pathways that promote HRS cell proliferation.[34] The most successful targeted therapy developed to date in HL has been brentuximab vedotin, an ADC directed against the CD30 receptor. Early clinical studies targeting CD30 with naked antibodies SGN-30 (cAC10), and MDX-060 did not demonstrate meaningful anti-tumor activity largely attributed to suboptimal antigen binding, and neutralization of anti CD30 antibodies by soluble CD30.[35,36,37] In an effort to increase cytotoxicity, a valine–citrulline peptide linker to monomethyl auristatin E, a synthetic analogue of the naturally occurring antimitotic agent dolastatin 10, was added to the chimeric antibody cAC10 (SGN-30) creating the ADC brentuximab vedotin. Robust antitumor activity reported in 2 phase I clinical trials led to a lot of hype regarding this agent.[38,39] These data were subsequently confirmed in a phase II pivotal trial of 102 patients with heavily pretreated HL who had relapsed after ASCT.[17] Overall treatment was well tolerated, and grade 3 or greater events or dose-limiting toxicities

Table 1
Current results in selected targeted therapies in HL

Drug/Phase	Main Target	Clinical Trial Number	Failed ASCT (%)	Clinical Results	Reference
Receptor Targeted Therapies					
SGN-30 (I)	CD 30+ HRS cells	NCT00051597	83[a]	No significant response	35,36,37
SGN-30 (II)		NCT00337194	68		
MDX-060 (1/2)	CD 30+ HRS cells	NCT00284804	87[a]	No significant response	35,36,37
BV					
BV(I)	CD 30+ HRS cells	NCT00947856	73[a]	PIVOTAL Trial: ORR 75%, CR 34%, median	17,38,39
BV(I)		NCT01100502	68[a]	PFS 5.6 mo, median DOR 20.5 mo	
BV(II)		NCT01060904	100	—	
HCD122 (II)	CD40+ HRS cells; Th2/Treg signaling	NCT00670592	NR	ORR 16% (all PR)	49
Galiximab (II)	CD80+ HRS cells	NCT00516217	83	ORR of 6.9%, TTP 1.6 mo	46,47
Microenvironment Targeting					
Lenalidomide (II)	Immunomodulation, antiangiogenesis	NCT00540007	76	ORR 19% (N = 32)	54,55
Lenalidomide (II)		NCT00478959	67	ORR 13% (N = 15)	
AFM 13 (I)	CD 16/30+ HRS cells	NCT01221571	NR	7% PR/50% SD	56
Rituximab single agent (I pilot)	CD20+ peritumoral B lymphocytes	—	82	ORR 22%, median DOR 8.7 mo	61,62,63,64
Rituximab + gemcitabine (II)	CD20+ HRS cells		55	ORR 48%, median FFS 2.7 mo	
Rituximab + ABVD frontline (I)		NCT00504504	0	EFS 83% and OS 96%	
Rituximab + ABVD frontline (II)		NCT00369681	0	EFS 83% and OS 98%	
PLX3397 (II)	CSF1R inhibitor	NCT01217229	NR	ORR 5%	66

Adoptive Immunotherapy					
EBV+ specific cytotoxic T cells	EBV+ HRS cells	NCT00058617[a]	40	83% of 28 patients with EBV+ HL had a clinical response, including 4 CRs sustained >9 mo	67,68
Downstream Signaling Pathway					
Panobinostat (I)	Histone modification	NCT00742027	100	ORR 27% including 4% CR, median PFS was 6.1 mo	78
Vorinostat (I)	Histone modification, STAT signaling (pSTAT6)	NCT00132028	44	ORR 4%	77
Mocetinostat (I)	Histone modification, STAT signaling	NCT00358982	84	ORR 21%	80
Everolimus (I)	PI3K signaling, mTOR, TNFR signaling	NCT01022996	84	ORR 47% 8 PR, 1 CR median TTP 7.2 mo, 4 responders remained progression free at 12 mo	88
SB1518	JAK/STAT pathway	NCT01263899	NR	No significant clinical activity	85

Abbreviations: ABVD, Adriamycin, bleomycin, vinblastine, and dacarbazine; BV, Brentuximab vedotin; DOR, duration of response; EBV, Epstein-Barr virus; EFS, event-free survival; FFS, failure-free survival; JAK, Janus kinase; mTOR, mammalian target of rapamycin; NA, not available; NR, not reported; ORR, overall response rate; PFS, progression-free survival; PI3K, phosphatidylinositol 3-kinase; PR, partial response; SD, stable disease; STAT, signal transducer and activator of transcription; Th2, T helper 2 cells; TNFR, tumor necrosis factor receptor; Treg, regulatory T cells; TTP, time to progression.
All trials are in relapsed/refractory patients unless otherwise indicated.
[a] Includes patients with HL and non-HL.

Table 2
Selected ongoing clinical trials of novel agents

Drug	Main Target	Clinical Trial Number
Receptor Targeted Therapies		
BV combinations		
Frontline		
Phase 3 frontline with AVD vs brentuximab/AVD	CD 30+ HRS cells	NCT01712490
ECAPP B vs ECADD B (frontline)		NCT01569204
Relapsed/Refractory		
ABVD → BV (relapsed)		NCT01578967
BV + bendamustine (relapsed)		NCT01874054
BV + ipilimumab (relapsed)		NCT01896999
BV vs ICE pre ASCT (relapsed)		NCT01393717
BV → ICE (relapsed)		NCT01508312
BV + rituximab (relapsed)		NCT01900496
Maintenance		
BV maintenance after ASCT (ATHERA) (maintenance)		NCT01620229
TNX-650	IL-13	NCT00441818
Microenvironment Targeting		
Lenalidomide Combinations (relapsed)		
AVD	Immunomodulation,	NCT01056679
Bendamustine	antiangiogenesis	NCT01412307
Romidepsin		NCT01742793
Everolimus		NCT01075321
Rituximab Combinations		
Frontline		
Rituximab ABVD vs ABVD phase 2	CD20+ peritumoral	NCT00654732
Rituximab + BEACOPP (HD18)	B lymphocytes;	NCT00515554
Relapsed	CD20+ HRS cells	
Rituximab + Bendamustine		NCT01900496
Ipilimumab (relapsed)	Immunomodulation of tumor microenvironment	NCT01896999
Nivolumab[a] (relapsed)	PD-1 expressing peritumoral lymphocytes	NCT01592370
CDX1127 (relapsed)	Anti-CD27 antibody	NCT01460134
Adoptive Immunotherapy		
Autologous CAR.CD30 EBV specific-cytotoxic T-lymphocytes (relapsed)	EBV+ CD30+ HRS cells; CD30+ HRS cells	NCT01192464
Downstream Signaling Pathways		
MLN4924 (relapsed)	NFκB via inhibition of Ned8	NCT00722488
Everolimus (relapsed)		
Everolimus and panobinostat	PI3K signaling, mTOR,	NCT00918333
Everolimus and lenalidomide	TNFR signaling	NCT01075321

Abbreviations: ABVD, Adriamycin, bleomycin, vinblastine, and dacarbazine; AVD, Adriamycin, vinblastine, dacarbazine; BEACOPP, bleomycin, etoposide, Adriamycin, cyclophosphamide, vincristine, procarbazine, and prednisone; BV, brentuximab vedotin; CAR, chimeric antigen receptor; DOR, duration of response; EBV, Epstein-Barr virus; ECADD B, etoposide, cyclophosphamide, Adriamycin, doxorubicin, dacarbazine, and brentuximab; ECAPP B, brentuximab vedotin in combination with etoposide, cyclophosphamide, Adriamycin, procarbazine, prednisone, and brentuximab; ICE, ifosfamide, carboplatinum, and etoposide; IL, interleukin; mTOR, mammalian target of rapamycin; NA, not available; NFκB, nuclear factor kappa B; NR, not reported; ORR, overall response rate; PD-1, programmed death-1; PFS, progression-free survival; PI3K, phosphatidylinositol 3-kinase; PR, partial response; TNFR, tumor necrosis factor receptor; TTP, time to progression.

[a] Includes patients with HL and non-HL.

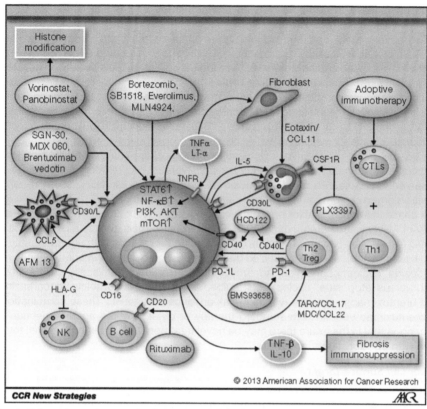

Fig. 1. Selected novel agents in the context of the biologic targets. CSF, colony-stimulating factor; mTOR, mammalian target of rapamycin; NK, natural killer; PI3K, phosphatidylinositol 3-kinase; TARC, thymus and activation-regulated chemokine; Th, T helper cells; TNFR, tumor necrosis factor receptor. AKT, protein kinase B; BMS93658, nivolumab; CCL, chemokine ligand; HCD122, lucatumumab; HLA-G, human leukocyte antigen G; LT, lymphotoxin; MDC, macrophage derived chemokine. (*Courtesy of* American Association for Cancer Research, with permission; *From* Diefenbach C, Steidl C. New strategies in Hodgkin lymphoma: better risk profiling and novel treatments. Clin Cancer Res 2013;19(11):2799, with permission.)

(DLT) included neutropenia (20%), thrombocytopenia (8%), peripheral sensory neuropathy (8%), and anemia (6%). The response rate in this heavily pretreated population was striking, with an overall response rate (ORR) of 75% and a CR rate of 34%. The median progression-free survival (PFS) was 5.6 months, with a median duration of response (DOR) of 20.5 months.[17]

These compelling data led to the Food and Drug Administration approval of brentuximab vedotin in 2011 for patients with relapsed/refractory HL who have failed ASCT or 2 chemotherapy regimens. Data also suggest that brentuximab vedotin is active as a retreatment strategy with an ORR of 57%.[40] Recently, 2 retrospective analyses suggest that brentuximab vedotin also provides a potential bridge to successful alloSCT.[41,42] The combination of brentuximab vedotin with donor lymphocyte infusion has been shown to induce both antitumor immunity and sustained clinical responses in 4 patients with early relapse after alloSCT.[43] Ongoing trials are evaluating brentuximab vedotin as a maintenance strategy for high-risk patients after ASCT and for relapsed disease in combination with chemotherapy or immune-based therapies, such as ipilimumab (see **Table 2**).

The development and subsequent approval of brentuximab vedotin is a clear example of a novel therapy that has moved well beyond hype and offers hope for patients with relapsed and refractory HL. As a logical next step, trials evaluating its role in the frontline setting are ongoing (see **Tables 1** and **2**). Preliminary results of a phase I trial evaluating the combination of brentuximab with doxorubicin hydrochloride (Adriamycin), bleomycin, vinblastine, and dacarbazine (ABVD) has been reported.[44] Unfortunately, 44% (11 out of 25) of patients experienced significant pulmonary toxicity, including 2 patients who died while on study. Subsequently, with modification to exclude bleomycin (Adriamycin, vinblastine, dacarbazine [AVD]), 7 of the 11 patients completed treatment without further toxicity. Notably, no pulmonary toxicity was observed in an expanded AVD-brentuximab cohort, and preliminary results report a positron emission tomography/computed tomography CR of 96%.[44] These data led to a phase III frontline trial for patients with untreated advanced HL evaluating the activity of ABVD versus brentuximab-AVD. Other frontline trials include a phase I trial of ABVD followed by 6 cycles of brentuximab vedotin for patients with untreated stage I and II nonbulky HL and a randomized trial of brentuximab vedotin in combination with etoposide, cyclophosphamide, Adriamycin, procarbazine, prednisone, and brentuximab versus etoposide, cyclophosphamide, Adriamycin, doxorubicin, dacarbazine, and brentuximab in patients with high-risk advanced-stage HL. These combinations of brentuximab vedotin with standard therapy or other targeted agents continue to offer hope that in the future there may be novel treatment platforms that are well tolerated with possibly superior activity.

Other Cell Surface Targets

CD80 is a costimulatory molecule highly expressed on HRS cells and inhibits antigen-specific T-cell lymphoproliferation and interferon-gamma secretion.[45] Galiximab, a primatized immunoglobulin G 1 monoclonal antibody against CD80, has high affinity binding for CD80 and induces antibody-dependent cytotoxicity (ADCC).[46] In a phase II clinical trial in patients with relapsed and refractory HL, galiximab was well tolerated but had disappointing activity, with an ORR of 6.9% and a median time to progression (TTP) of 1.6 months.[46,47]

CD40 is widely expressed on B and T cells and a member of the TNF receptor family, which induces cell proliferation, survival, secretion of cytokines, and activation of both the classic (canonical) and alternative (noncanonical) pathways of nuclear factor kappa B (NFκB) signaling.[48] Lucatumumab (HCD122) targets both CD40+ HRS cells and Th2/Treg signaling and has been investigated in HL. A phase II trial reported an ORR of 16%, all partial responses (PRs) in 18 patients with relapsed/refractory HL.[49] The therapy was generally well tolerated, and reversible asymptomatic hepatotoxicity was the primary DLT.

Agents that have been investigated but are not currently in development include antibodies to the TRAIL protein and CD25, the alpha chain of the IL-2 receptor. A phase I trial of the TRAIL-R2 antibody AMG655 in combination with bortezomib or vorinostat was suspended because of poor patient accrual. A clinical trial of the anti-CD25 ricin A-chain immunotoxin RFT5-SPMT-dgA had significant toxicity caused by vascular leak syndrome and disappointing results, with only 13% of patients achieving a PR.[50] A monoclonal antibody targeting IL-13 (TNX-650) is currently under investigation; however, to date, no clinical data have been reported.

In summary, although there has been considerable hype based on the biologic rationale of using antibodies to target differentially expressed cell-surface receptors, none have matched the efficacy of brentuximab vedotin. More insightful science and combination strategies are required to truly translate to hope in the clinical setting.

TARGETING THE TUMOR MICROENVIRONMENT

Monotherapies targeting only the HRS cells are limited in their efficacy because of the major role of the microenvironment in regulating HRS function and survival.[19]

Strategies targeting tumor-microenvironment interactions aim to disrupt its cellular components or activate peritumoral T and natural killer (NK) cells to induce antitumor responses. Encouraging preclinical data of agents in development include immunomodulatory drugs (lenalidomide); monoclonal-antibody directed targeting of peritumoral CD20-positive B cells (rituximab, alemtuzumab); bispecific antibodies, such as AFM13, which simultaneously targets CD30 bearing HRS cells and CD16 on NK cells; selective inhibition of colony-stimulating factor-1 (CSF1R), a growth factor for TAMs; the anti-CTLA-4 antibody ipilimumab; and the checkpoint inhibitors targeting PD-1 and anti-PDL-1.[51,52] Ongoing trials are outlined in **Table 2**.

Lenalidomide is an immunomodulatory and antiangiogenic agent, with a putative mechanism of activating CTLs and NK cells against HRS cells.[53] The safety and efficacy of lenalidomide as a monotherapy has been investigated in several studies. In a multicenter phase II study, 36 patients with relapsed HL were treated with 25 mg/d of lenalidomide on days 1 to 21 of a 28-day cycle. The ORR was 19%, with moderate grade 3 to 4 hematologic toxicity noted: neutropenia (47%), leukopenia (29%), anemia (26%), and thrombocytopenia (18%).[54] A smaller study of 15 patients reported similar results for toxicity as well as efficacy with an ORR of 13%. Seven additional patients had stable disease. The median TTP was 3.2 months.[55] Cumulatively, these studies suggest that lenalidomide has modest single-agent activity in relapsed HL. There is hope that efficacy may be enhanced by combinations with chemotherapy or other HRS-targeting agents with trials ongoing (see **Table 2**).

AFM13, a bispecific tetravalent human antibody construct that simultaneously targets CD30 and CD16 on NK cells, has been evaluated in a phase I clinical trial in relapsed/refractory HL. Patients were heavily pretreated with a median of 6 (range 3–11) prior therapies. Of the 28 patients enrolled, 9 had received previous brentuximab vedotin and 14 were refractory to prior therapy. AFM13 was safe and well tolerated. The most frequent adverse events included infusion-related reactions (headache, fever, fatigue, and myalgia) in 33% of patients. Moderate clinical activity (2 patients achieved PRs, 14 patients with stable disease (SD)) was demonstrated, and more mature follow-up is needed to discern the potential.[56]

Although HRS cells rarely express CD20, the tumor microenvironment is rich in CD20-expressing B cells; a study suggests that circulating clonotypic B cells may be the HL tumor initiating cells.[57] Some studies suggest that these B cells deliver survival signals to HRS cells and suppress T-cell activation via IL-10 production.[58] In contrast, other studies report that the presence of CD20-expressing B cells in the tumor microenvironment is associated with improved survival.[59,60] Nonetheless, targeting CD20 with the monoclonal antibody rituximab has been actively investigated. In a pilot study, 22 patients with relapsed/refractory HL were treated with single-agent rituximab. The ORR was 22% and included PRs as well as CRs.[61] Six of 7 patients with CD20-negative HRS cells experienced resolution of B symptoms, suggesting a possible role for CD20-positive B cells in mediating the systemic cytokine response.[61] Therefore, it is unclear whether the activity of rituximab is caused by a direct effect on HRS cells (that are occasionally CD20 positive) or a depletion of supporting B cells and peritumoral CD20-positive cells. These encouraging single-agent data provided the rationale to investigate rituximab in combination with chemotherapy. The safety and efficacy of rituximab and gemcitabine was investigated in 33 patients with relapsed HL. The ORR was 48% independent of HRS cell CD20 expression; however, the median failure-free survival was only 2.7 months.[62] Two phase II trials have evaluated rituximab in combination with ABVD. In the first trial, 78 patients with newly diagnosed HL were treated with weekly rituximab for 6 weeks and standard ABVD for 6 cycles.[63] The combination was well tolerated, with neutropenia, fatigue, and nausea being the most frequent treatment-related adverse events. At 68 months, the event-free survival (EFS) and OS were 83% and 96%, respectively. These results were superior to ABVD alone when compared with institutional historical data. A second phase II study reported similar results, with a 3-year EFS and OS of 83% and 98%, respectively.[64] In this study, circulating clonotypic B cells were associated with a greater frequency of relapse. Other ongoing studies are evaluating the contribution of rituximab to first line augmented bleomycin, etoposide, Adriamycin, cyclophosphamide, vincristine, procarbazine, and prednisone for patients with advanced untreated HL (HD18) and in combination with ABVD as a frontline therapy for patients with advanced-stage poor-risk HL (see **Table 2**).

In summary, although there is reasonable hype about the rationale to target CD20, the results of randomized controlled trials are required before the question of hype versus hope can be definitively answered.

CD52 is another cell-surface receptor highly expressed on peritumoral B cells. Alemtuzumab, a humanized monoclonal anti-CD52 antibody, binds to CD52 purportedly inducing cell lysis via ADCC.[65] A phase II study investigating the efficacy of single-agent alemtuzumab in relapsed/refractory HL was terminated because of slow patient accrual, and data have not been reported to date. The efficacy of the combination of alemtuzumab with etoposide, prednisone, vincristine, cyclophosphamide, and Adriamycin chemotherapy in relapsed/refractory HL is currently under investigation (see **Table 2**).

Direct immune-based approaches, which reverse the anergy of peritumoral T cells and stimulate antitumor cytolytic activity, represent another novel strategy against relapsed/refractory HL. The association of the high expression of TAMs with a short PFS led to significant hype for evaluating their inhibition with compound PLX3397, a selective inhibitor of CSF1R (a growth factor for TAMs). Unfortunately, despite the inhibition of both CSF1R and Kit, in a phase II trial of 20 patients with heavily pretreated HL, PLX3397 had only modest activity, with an ORR of 5% and a median PFS of 56 days.[66] Therefore, the role of CSF1R in HL lymphoma biology needs to be better understood before these strategies move from hype into hope.

Lastly, immune-activating strategies, such as the combination of the anti-CTLA-4 antibody (ipilimumab) with brentuximab vedotin and the anti-CD27 antibody (CDX1127), are being investigated. Checkpoint inhibitors against PD-1 expressed on peritumoral T cells or PDL-1 expressed on the HRS cell surface are also undergoing active investigation (see **Table 2**).

In summary, it is too early in development to discern whether the data from agents targeting reactive immune cells in the tumor microenvironment, as summarized in this section, will translate to hope. Results of ongoing clinical trials over the next few years will help shed some light on the efficacy of these agents both in terms of a response rate and durability.

ADOPTIVE IMMUNOTHERAPY IN HL

Adoptive immunotherapy allows the generation and transfer of T cells engineered ex vivo to target and attack tumor cells in the host as well as immune activation of the tumor microenvironment. In relapsed/refractory Epstein-Barr virus positive (EBV+) HL, an adoptive approach using ex vivo expansion of viral EBV antigen-specific CTLs produced striking results, albeit in a small number of patients.[67,68] In this pilot study, 83% (5 of 6) patients with relapsed EBV+ HL had a clinical response, of which 4 achieved CRs sustained for more than 9 months. Other trials of adoptive immunotherapy (ie, targeting EBV-HL through MAGE antigen or genetically engineered T lymphocytes expressing a chimeric CD30 antigen receptor) are ongoing but have not reported data to date.[69,70] Only time will tell if these innovative strategies will constitute a new domain of hope or not.

TARGETING DOWNSTREAM SIGNALING AND INTRACELLULAR SURVIVAL PATHWAYS

Several drugs target constitutively activated downstream signaling pathways that drive HRS cell proliferation and enhance tumor cell survival. Epigenetic changes in HRS cells modulate B-cell silencing, immune escape, and the transcription of genes underlying cell proliferation and survival.[71] The acetylation state of proteins are modified by the opposing effects of both histone acetyltransferases and histone deacetylases (HDACs). There are currently 4 classes of HDACs: classes I and IV are constitutive nuclear proteins that regulate cell proliferation, class II regulate genes that promote cell growth and shuttle between the nucleus and the cytoplasm, and class III regulate chromatin structure.[72] Increased expression of HDACs relative to normal tissues has been observed in HL and, in at least one study, correlated with a poor treatment outcome.[73]

Histone deacetylase inhibitors (HDACI) modulate cellular processes and signaling pathways that are dysregulated in cancers.[74,75] HDACI target tumor cells and their interaction with their local microenvironment through multiple epigenetic mechanisms, including chromatin condensation and acetylation of histones affecting gene expression. Treatment of patients with HL with HDACI decreases the secretion of the inhibitory cytokine CCL17 (TARC) in vitro.[76] Currently, 2 broad classes of HDACIs are under investigation in HL: pan HDAC inhibitors that inhibit HDAC class I and II (ie, vorinostat and panobinostat) and selective HDACIs that preferentially inhibit class I HDACs (mocetinostat and etinostat).

Vorinostat, mocetinostat, and panobinostat have been investigated as monotherapies in relapsed/refractory HL. In a phase II study of oral vorinostat, the ORR was only 4%.[77] More promising reports have been reported for panobinostat in a phase II trial of 129 patients with HL, all of whom had failed ASCT. The primary toxicities were hematologic. Grade 3 to 4 toxicities included 79% thrombocytopenia, 21% anemia, and 21% neutropenia. The ORR in this heavily pretreated patient population was 27% (23% PR, 4% CR), with a median DOR of 6.9 months and an estimated 1-year OS rate of 78%. The median PFS was approximately 6 months, and 52 patients (40%) had PFS greater than 24 weeks.[78] Responses were associated with a decrease in serum TARC levels.[78,79]

Mocetinostat has been evaluated in a phase 2 trial in relapsed/refractory HL. Significant toxicity was seen at the 110 mg dose including grade 3 or greater myelosuppression, fatigue, pneumonia, and pleural effusions in 4 patients (3 ≥grade 3). The drug was better tolerated at the reduced dose of 85 mg, with an ORR of 21%.[80]

Cumulatively, these data suggest that HDACI have activity; however, the hematologic toxicity profile will likely make combination strategies with chemotherapy challenging. Currently, the optimal HDACI strategy to move these drugs from the hype category to the hope category remains unclear.

HRS cells constitutively express NFκB, in part as a result of somatic mutations in pathway members and regulators, as well as other antiapoptotic proteins, which inhibit both the intrinsic and extrinsic pathways of apoptosis.[21,23] Bortezomib, a reversible proteasome inhibitor of NFκB signaling, enhances apoptosis through down-regulation of the antiapoptotic molecules X-linked inhibitor of apotosis protein and cellular FLICE-like inhibitory protein, and has a putative role as a chemotherapy sensitizing agent.[81] Although bortezomib demonstrated antiproliferative activity in vitro, a phase II clinical trial in relapsed/refractory HL failed to demonstrate meaningful clinical activity.[82] The evidence for synergy between cytotoxic chemotherapy and bortezomib in non-HL led to the evaluation of the combination of bortezomib and chemotherapy in relapsed/refractory HL. In a phase I trial of ifosfamide, carboplatinum, and etoposide (ICE) in combination with bortezomib (BICE) given on days 1 and 4 of standard infusion, the ORR for 12 patients was 69%, but significant myelosuppression was seen.[83] A second study combined bortezomib given twice weekly (days 1, 4, 8, 11) in a 3-week cycle at a dose of 1 mg/m^2 with gemcitabine 800 mg/m^2 on days 1 and 8. This combination had significantly lower activity (ORR 22%) with higher toxicity (grade 3 transaminitis) than the BICE-treated patients and was not pursued further. A study targeting NFκB with MLN4924, a small molecule inhibitor of neddylation 8, has recently been terminated because of slow accrual, and no data have been reported to date.

Other constitutively activated pathways in HRS cells include Janus kinase-STAT (JAK-STAT) and the phosphatidylinositol 3-kinase pathway (PI3K/AKT/mammalian target of rapamycin [mTOR] pathway). Inhibitors of JAK2 inhibitors suppress STAT phosphorylation in HL cells lines and downregulate the expression of PDL-1 in vitro[84]; however, a phase I trial of the JAK2 inhibitor SB1518 did not have significant clinical activity despite a tolerable safety profile.[85]

Inhibition of MTOR has a myriad of in vitro effects, including enhancement of apoptosis, cell cycle arrest, and autophagy.[86,87] The clinical activity of the MTOR inhibitor everolimus was evaluated in a phase II trial in patients with relapsed/refractory HL. The ORR of this heavily pretreated patient population was 47%, with 8 patients achieving a PR and one a CR. The median TTP was 7.2 months, with 4 responders remaining progression free at 12 months.[88] Overall, the therapy was reasonably well tolerated, except in 4 patients who experienced grade 3 or greater pulmonary toxicity. A synergy between targeting MTOR and other inhibitors of downstream signaling, such as PI3K and HDAC, has been suggested by in vitro data; this combination is currently being evaluated. In a phase I/II study of the combination of everolimus with the HDACI panobinostat, the ORR for 13 patients with HL was 46%.[89] Combinations of everolimus with immunomodulatory agents, such as lenalidomide, as well as with PI3K inhibitors are currently under investigation.

SUMMARY

Advances in HL biology over the past few years have yielded a plethora of novel targets and an unprecedented opportunity to develop newer therapies. These targeted therapies offer the potential to increase cure rates in patients with relapsed and refractory HL, along with the hope of decreasing long-term toxicity. The approval of brentuximab vedotin clearly offers new hope to patients with relapsed and refractory disease and may have promise as a frontline therapy. Currently, there are many novel targeted therapies under clinical investigation in HL and many more waiting to move from bench to bedside. Although these advances are exciting, it is unlikely that one size will fit all or that any single therapy or therapeutic platform will be curative for all patients. The challenges ahead are to identify strategies that offer maximal tumor eradication with minimal systemic toxicity and to identify subsets of patients with the highest likelihood of efficacy to a particular therapy. To accomplish this, more robust methods of risk stratification incorporating both clinical and biologic factors to identify patients at the highest risk of therapy failure are needed. This gap needs to be addressed before the full potential of novel targeted therapies can be realized, and the hope of customized targeted therapies will then surpass the hype.

REFERENCES

1. American Cancer Society. Cancer facts and figures 2013. Atlanta (GA): American Cancer Society; 2013.
2. Available at: http://seer.cancer.gov/statfacts/html/hodg.html. Accessed August 20, 2013.
3. Koontz MZ, Horning SJ, Balise R, et al. Risk of therapy-related secondary leukemia in Hodgkin lymphoma: the Stanford University experience over three generations of clinical trials. J Clin Oncol 2013;31(5):592–8.
4. De Bruin ML, Sparidans J, van't Veer MB, et al. Breast cancer risk in female survivors of Hodgkin's lymphoma: lower risk after smaller radiation volumes. J Clin Oncol 2009;27(26):4239–46.
5. Hodgson DC. Late effects in the era of modern therapy for Hodgkin lymphoma. Hematology Am Soc Hematol Educ Program 2011;2011:323–9.
6. Gordon LI, Hong F, Fisher RI, et al. Randomized phase III trial of ABVD versus Stanford V with or without radiation therapy in locally extensive and advanced-stage Hodgkin lymphoma: an intergroup study coordinated by the Eastern Cooperative Oncology Group (E2496). J Clin Oncol 2013;31(6):684–91.
7. Engert A, Haverkamp H, Kobe C, et al. Reduced-intensity chemotherapy and PET-guided radiotherapy in patients with advanced stage Hodgkin's lymphoma (HD15 trial): a randomised, open-label, phase 3 non-inferiority trial. Lancet 2012;379(9828):1791–9.
8. Schmitz N, Pfistner B, Sextro M, et al. Aggressive conventional chemotherapy compared with high-dose chemotherapy with autologous haemopoietic stem-cell transplantation for relapsed chemosensitive Hodgkin's disease: a randomised trial. Lancet 2002;359(9323):2065–71.
9. Moskowitz CH, Nimer SD, Zelenetz AD, et al. A 2-step comprehensive high-dose chemoradiotherapy second-line program for relapsed and refractory Hodgkin disease: analysis by intent to treat and development of a prognostic model. Blood 2001;97(3):616–23.
10. von Tresckow B, Engert A. The emerging role of PET in Hodgkin lymphoma patients receiving autologous stem cell transplant. Expert Rev Hematol 2012;5(5): 483–6.
11. Horning SJ, Chao NJ, Negrin RS, et al. High-dose therapy and autologous hematopoietic progenitor cell transplantation for recurrent or refractory Hodgkin's disease: analysis of the Stanford University results and prognostic indices. Blood 1997;89(3):801–13.
12. Brice P, Bouabdallah R, Moreau P, et al. Prognostic factors for survival after high-dose therapy and autologous stem cell transplantation for patients with relapsing Hodgkin's disease: analysis of 280 patients from the French registry. Societe Francaise de Greffe de Moelle. Bone Marrow Transplant 1997;20(1):21–6.
13. Sureda A, Constans M, Iriondo A, et al. Prognostic factors affecting long-term outcome after stem cell transplantation in Hodgkin's lymphoma autografted after a first relapse. Ann Oncol 2005;16(4):625–33.

14. Josting A, Franklin J, May M, et al. New prognostic score based on treatment outcome of patients with relapsed Hodgkin's lymphoma registered in the database of the German Hodgkin's lymphoma study group. J Clin Oncol 2002;20(1):221–30.

15. Arai S, Fanale M, Devos S, et al. Defining a Hodgkin lymphoma population for novel therapeutics after relapse from autologous hematopoietic cell transplant. Leuk Lymphoma 2013;54(11):2531–3.

16. Thomson KJ, Peggs KS, Smith P, et al. Superiority of reduced-intensity allogeneic transplantation over conventional treatment for relapse of Hodgkin's lymphoma following autologous stem cell transplantation. Bone Marrow Transplant 2008;41(9):765–70.

17. Younes A, Gopal AK, Smith SE, et al. Results of a pivotal phase II study of brentuximab vedotin for patients with relapsed or refractory Hodgkin's lymphoma. J Clin Oncol 2012;30(18):2183–9.

18. Aldinucci D, Gloghini A, Pinto A, et al. The classical Hodgkin's lymphoma microenvironment and its role in promoting tumour growth and immune escape. J Pathol 2010;221(3):248–63.

19. Steidl C, Connors JM, Gascoyne RD. Molecular pathogenesis of Hodgkin's lymphoma: increasing evidence of the importance of the microenvironment. J Clin Oncol 2011;29(14):1812–26.

20. Hsi ED. Biologic features of Hodgkin lymphoma and the development of biologic prognostic factors in Hodgkin lymphoma: tumor and microenvironment. Leuk Lymphoma 2008;49(9):1668–80.

21. Kuppers R. The biology of Hodgkin's lymphoma. Nat Rev Cancer 2009;9(1):15–27.

22. Khan G. Epstein-Barr virus, cytokines, and inflammation: a cocktail for the pathogenesis of Hodgkin's lymphoma? Exp Hematol 2006;34(4):399–406.

23. Farrell K, Jarrett RF. The molecular pathogenesis of Hodgkin lymphoma. Histopathology 2011;58(1):15–25.

24. Kim LH, Eow GI, Peh SC, et al. The role of CD30, CD40 and CD95 in the regulation of proliferation and apoptosis in classical Hodgkin's lymphoma. Pathology 2003;35(5):428–35.

25. Yamamoto R, Nishikori M, Kitawaki T, et al. PD-1-PD-1 ligand interaction contributes to immunosuppressive microenvironment of Hodgkin lymphoma. Blood 2008;111(6):3220–4.

26. Green MR, Monti S, Rodig SJ, et al. Integrative analysis reveals selective 9p24.1 amplification, increased PD-1 ligand expression, and further induction via JAK2 in nodular sclerosing Hodgkin lymphoma and primary mediastinal large B-cell lymphoma. Blood 2010;116(17):3268–77.

27. Gandhi MK, Moll G, Smith C, et al. Galectin-1 mediated suppression of Epstein-Barr virus specific T-cell immunity in classic Hodgkin lymphoma. Blood 2007;110(4):1326–9.

28. Juszczynski P, Ouyang J, Monti S, et al. The AP1-dependent secretion of galectin-1 by Reed Sternberg cells fosters immune privilege in classical Hodgkin lymphoma. Proc Natl Acad Sci U S A 2007;104(32):13134–9.

29. van den Berg A, Visser L, Poppema S. High expression of the CC chemokine TARC in Reed-Sternberg cells. A possible explanation for the characteristic T-cell infiltratein Hodgkin's lymphoma. Am J Pathol 1999;154(6):1685–91.

30. Aldinucci D, Lorenzon D, Cattaruzza L, et al. Expression of CCR5 receptors on Reed-Sternberg cells and Hodgkin lymphoma cell lines: involvement of

CCL5/Rantes in tumor cell growth and microenvironmental interactions. Int J Cancer 2008;122(4):769–76.

31. Cattaruzza L, Gloghini A, Olivo K, et al. Functional coexpression of Interleukin (IL)-7 and its receptor (IL-7R) on Hodgkin and Reed-Sternberg cells: Involvement of IL-7 in tumor cell growth and microenvironmental interactions of Hodgkin's lymphoma. Int J Cancer 2009;125(5):1092–101.

32. Sauer M, Plutschow A, Jachimowicz RD, et al. Baseline serum TARC levels predict therapy outcome in patients with Hodgkin lymphoma. Am J Hematol 2013; 88(2):113–5.

33. Tan KL, Scott DW, Hong F, et al. Tumor-associated macrophages predict inferior outcomes in classic Hodgkin lymphoma: a correlative study from the E2496 Intergroup trial. Blood 2012;120(16):3280–7.

34. Zheng B, Fiumara P, Li YV, et al. MEK/ERK pathway is aberrantly active in Hodgkin disease: a signaling pathway shared by CD30, CD40, and RANK that regulates cell proliferation and survival. Blood 2003;102(3):1019–27.

35. Ansell SM, Horwitz SM, Engert A, et al. Phase I/II study of an anti-CD30 monoclonal antibody (MDX-060) in Hodgkin's lymphoma and anaplastic large-cell lymphoma. J Clin Oncol 2007;25(19):2764–9.

36. Forero-Torres A, Leonard JP, Younes A, et al. A Phase II study of SGN-30 (anti-CD30 mAb) in Hodgkin lymphoma or systemic anaplastic large cell lymphoma. Br J Haematol 2009;146(2):171–9.

37. Blum KA, Jung SH, Johnson JL, et al. Serious pulmonary toxicity in patients with Hodgkin's lymphoma with SGN-30, gemcitabine, vinorelbine, and liposomal doxorubicin is associated with an FcgammaRIIIa-158 V/F polymorphism. Ann Oncol 2010;21(11):2246–54.

38. Younes A, Bartlett NL, Leonard JP, et al. Brentuximab vedotin (SGN-35) for relapsed CD30-positive lymphomas. N Engl J Med 2010;363(19):1812–21.

39. Fanale MA, Forero-Torres A, Rosenblatt JD, et al. A Phase I Weekly Dosing Study of Brentuximab Vedotin in Patients with Relapsed/Refractory CD30-Positive Hematologic Malignancies. Clin Cancer Res 2012;18(1):248–55.

40. Bartlett N, Brice P, Chen RW, et al. Retreatment with brentuximab vedotin in CD30–positive hematologic malignancies: a phase II study. ASCO Annual Meeting Abstracts. J Clin Oncol 2012;30(Suppl) [abstract 8027].

41. Chen R, Palmer JM, Thomas SH, et al. Brentuximab vedotin enables successful reduced-intensity allogeneic hematopoietic cell transplantation in patients with relapsed or refractory Hodgkin lymphoma. Blood 2012;119(26):6379–81.

42. Gibb A, Jones C, Bloor A, et al. Brentuximab vedotin in refractory CD30+ lymphomas: a bridge to allogeneic transplantation in approximately one quarter of patients treated on a named patient programme at a single UK center. Haematologica 2013;98(4):611–4.

43. Theurich S, Malcher J, Wennhold K, et al. Brentuximab vedotin combined with donor lymphocyte infusions for early relapse of Hodgkin lymphoma after allogeneic stem-cell transplantation induces tumor-specific immunity and sustained clinical remission. J Clin Oncol 2013;31(5):e59–63.

44. Ansell SM, Connors JM, Park SI, et al. Frontline therapy with brentuximab vedotin combined with ABVD or AVD in patients with newly diagnosed advanced stage Hodgkin lymphoma. ASH Annual Meeting Abstracts 2012; 120(21):798.

45. Fleischer J, Soeth E, Reiling N, et al. Differential expression and function of CD80 (B7-1) and CD86 (B7-2) on human peripheral blood monocytes. Immunology 1996;89(4):592–8.

46. Smith SM, Schoder H, Johnson JL, et al. The anti-CD80 primatized monoclonal antibody, galiximab, is well-tolerated but has limited activity in relapsed Hodgkin lymphoma: CALGB 50602 (Alliance). Leuk Lymphoma 2013;54(7):1405–10.
47. Nozawa Y, Wakasa H, Abe M. Costimulatory molecules (CD80 and CD86) on Reed-Sternberg cells are associated with the proliferation of background T cells in Hodgkin's disease. Pathol Int 1998;48(1):10–4.
48. Aldinucci D, Gloghini A, Pinto A, et al. The role of CD40/CD40L and interferon regulatory factor 4 in Hodgkin lymphoma microenvironment. Leuk Lymphoma 2012;53(2):195–201.
49. Freedman AS, Kuruvilla J, Assouline SE, et al. Clinical activity of lucatumumab (HCD122) in patients (pts) with relapsed/refractory Hodgkin or non-Hodgkin lymphoma treated in a phase Ia/II clinical trial (NCT00670592). ASH Annual Meeting Abstracts 2010;116(21):284.
50. Engert A, Diehl V, Schnell R, et al. A phase-I study of an anti-CD25 ricin A-chain immunotoxin (RFT5-SMPT-dgA) in patients with refractory Hodgkin's lymphoma. Blood 1997;89(2):403–10.
51. Green MR, Rodig S, Juszczynski P, et al. Constitutive AP-1 activity and EBV infection induce PD-L1 in Hodgkin lymphomas and posttransplant lymphoproliferative disorders: implications for targeted therapy. Clin Cancer Res 2012;18(6):1611–8.
52. Steidl C, Diepstra A, Lee T, et al. Gene expression profiling of microdissected Hodgkin Reed-Sternberg cells correlates with treatment outcome in classical Hodgkin lymphoma. Blood 2012;120(17):3530–40.
53. Zhu D, Corral LG, Fleming YW, et al. Immunomodulatory drugs Revlimid (lenalidomide) and CC-4047 induce apoptosis of both hematological and solid tumor cells through NK cell activation. Cancer Immunol Immunother 2008;57(12):1849–59.
54. Fehniger TA, Larson S, Trinkaus K, et al. A phase 2 multicenter study of lenalidomide in relapsed or refractory classical Hodgkin lymphoma. Blood 2011;118(19):5119–25.
55. Kuruvilla J, Taylor D, Wang L, et al. Phase II trial of lenalidomide in patients with relapsed or refractory Hodgkin lymphoma. ASH Annual Meeting Abstracts 2008;112(11):3052.
56. Rothe A, Younes A, Reiners KS, et al. A phase I study with the bispecific anti-CD30 x anti-CD16A antibody construct AFM13 in patients with relapsed or refractory Hodgkin lymphoma. ASH Annual Meeting Abstracts 2011;118(21):3709.
57. Jones RJ, Gocke CD, Kasamon YL, et al. Circulating clonotypic B cells in classic Hodgkin lymphoma. Blood 2009;113(23):5920–6.
58. Banerjee D. Recent advances in the pathobiology of Hodgkin's lymphoma: potential impact on diagnostic, predictive, and therapeutic strategies. Adv Hematol 2011;2011:439456.
59. Chetaille B, Bertucci F, Finetti P, et al. Molecular profiling of classical Hodgkin lymphoma tissues uncovers variations in the tumor microenvironment and correlations with EBV infection and outcome. Blood 2009;113(12):2765–3775.
60. Steidl C, Lee T, Shah SP, et al. Tumor-associated macrophages and survival in classic Hodgkin's lymphoma. N Engl J Med 2010;362(10):875–85.
61. Younes A, Romaguera J, Hagemeister F, et al. A pilot study of rituximab in patients with recurrent, classic Hodgkin disease. Cancer 2003;98(2):310–4.
62. Oki Y, Pro B, Fayad LE, et al. Phase 2 study of gemcitabine in combination with rituximab in patients with recurrent or refractory Hodgkin lymphoma. Cancer 2008;112(4):831–6.

63. Younes A, Oki Y, McLaughlin P, et al. Phase 2 study of rituximab plus ABVD in patients with newly diagnosed classical Hodgkin lymphoma. Blood 2012; 119(18):4123–8.
64. Kasamon YL, Jacene HA, Gocke CD, et al. Phase 2 study of rituximab-ABVD in classical Hodgkin lymphoma. Blood 2012;119(18):4129–32.
65. Golay J, Manganini M, Rambaldi A, et al. Effect of alemtuzumab on neoplastic B cells. Haematologica 2004;89(12):1476–83.
66. Moskowitz CH, Younes A, de Vos S, et al. CSF1R Inhibition by PLX3397 in patients with relapsed or refractory Hodgkin lymphoma: results from a phase 2 single agent clinical trial. ASH Annual Meeting Abstracts 2012;120(21):1638.
67. Bollard CM, Gottschalk S, Leen AM, et al. Complete responses of relapsed lymphoma following genetic modification of tumor-antigen presenting cells and T-lymphocyte transfer. Blood 2007;110(8):2838–45.
68. Bollard CM, Aguilar L, Straathof KC, et al. Cytotoxic T lymphocyte therapy for Epstein-Barr virus+ Hodgkin's disease. J Exp Med 2004;200(12):1623–33.
69. Cruz CR, Gerdemann U, Leen AM, et al. Improving T-cell therapy for relapsed EBV-negative Hodgkin lymphoma by targeting upregulated MAGE-A4. Clin Cancer Res 2011;17(22):7058–66.
70. Di Stasi A, De Angelis B, Rooney CM, et al. T lymphocytes coexpressing CCR4 and a chimeric antigen receptor targeting CD30 have improved homing and antitumor activity in a Hodgkin tumor model. Blood 2009;113(25):6392–402.
71. Ushmorov A, Leithauser F, Sakk O, et al. Epigenetic processes play a major role in B-cell-specific gene silencing in classical Hodgkin lymphoma. Blood 2006; 107(6):2493–500.
72. Glozak MA, Seto E. Histone deacetylases and cancer. Oncogene 2007;26(37): 5420–32.
73. Adams H, Fritzsche FR, Dirnhofer S, et al. Class I histone deacetylases 1, 2 and 3 are highly expressed in classical Hodgkin's lymphoma. Expert Opin Ther Targets 2010;14(6):577–84.
74. Piekarz RL, Bates SE. Epigenetic modifiers: basic understanding and clinical development. Clin Cancer Res 2009;15(12):3918–26.
75. Sambucetti LC, Fischer DD, Zabludoff S, et al. Histone deacetylase inhibition selectively alters the activity and expression of cell cycle proteins leading to specific chromatin acetylation and antiproliferative effects. J Biol Chem 1999; 274(49):34940–7.
76. Buglio D, Georgakis GV, Hanabuchi S, et al. Vorinostat inhibits STAT6-mediated TH2 cytokine and TARC production and induces cell death in Hodgkin lymphoma cell lines. Blood 2008;112(4):1424–33.
77. Kirschbaum MH, Goldman BH, Zain JM, et al. A phase 2 study of vorinostat for treatment of relapsed or refractory Hodgkin lymphoma: Southwest Oncology Group Study S0517. Leuk Lymphoma 2012;53(2):259–62.
78. Younes A, Sureda A, Ben-Yehuda D, et al. Panobinostat in patients with relapsed/refractory Hodgkin's lymphoma after autologous stem-cell transplantation: results of a phase II study. J Clin Oncol 2012;30(18):2197–203.
79. Harrison SJ, Hsu AK, Neeson P, et al. Early thymus and activation-regulated chemokine (TARC) reduction and response following panobinostat treatment in patients with relapsed/refractory Hodgkin lymphoma following autologous stem cell transplant. Leuk Lymphoma 2013. [Epub ahead of print].
80. Younes A, Oki Y, Bociek RG, et al. Mocetinostat for relapsed classical Hodgkin's lymphoma: an open-label, single-arm, phase 2 trial. Lancet Oncol 2011;12(13): 1222–8.

81. Kashkar H, Deggerich A, Seeger JM, et al. NF-kappaB-independent down-regulation of XIAP by bortezomib sensitizes HL B cells against cytotoxic drugs. Blood 2007;109(9):3982–8.

82. Blum KA, Johnson JL, Niedzwiecki D, et al. Single agent bortezomib in the treatment of relapsed and refractory Hodgkin lymphoma: cancer and leukemia Group B protocol 50206. Leuk Lymphoma 2007;48(7):1313–9.

83. Fanale M, Fayad L, Pro B, et al. Phase I study of bortezomib plus ICE (BICE) for the treatment of relapsed/refractory Hodgkin lymphoma. Br J Haematol 2011; 154(2):284–6.

84. Derenzini E, Lemoine M, Buglio D, et al. The JAK inhibitor AZD1480 regulates proliferation and immunity in Hodgkin lymphoma. Blood Cancer J 2011;1(12): e46.

85. Younes A, Romaguera J, Fanale M, et al. Phase I study of a novel oral Janus kinase 2 inhibitor, SB1518, in patients with relapsed lymphoma: evidence of clinical and biologic activity in multiple lymphoma subtypes. J Clin Oncol 2012; 30(33):4161–7.

86. Witzig TE, Kaufmann SH. Inhibition of the phosphatidylinositol 3-kinase/mammalian target of rapamycin pathway in hematologic malignancies. Curr Treat Options Oncol 2006;7(4):285–94.

87. Rosich L, Colomer D, Roue G. Autophagy controls everolimus (RAD001) activity in mantle cell lymphoma. Autophagy 2013;9(1):115–7.

88. Johnston PB, Inwards DJ, Colgan JP, et al. A phase II trial of the oral mTOR inhibitor everolimus in relapsed Hodgkin lymphoma. Am J Hematol 2010;85(5): 320–4.

89. Younes A, Copeland A, Fanale MA, et al. Safety and efficacy of the novel combination of panobinostat (LBH589) and everolimus (RAD001) in relapsed/refractory Hodgkin and non-Hodgkin lymphoma. ASH Annual Meeting Abstracts 2011;118(21):3718.

Relapsed/Refractory Hodgkin Lymphoma

What Is the Best Salvage Therapy and Do We Need RIC-AlloSCT?

Mark Hertzberg, MBBS, PhD, FRACP, FRCPA

KEYWORDS

- Prognostic factors • Salvage chemotherapy • Autologous transplant
- FDG-PET scan • RIC-alloSCT

KEY POINTS

- For RR-HL, standard therapy consists of salvage chemotherapy followed by HDCT/ASCT + RT.
- Key adverse risk factors present at relapse/progression include short response duration <12 months, B symptoms, extranodal disease, as well as advanced stage and anemia.
- There is no obvious superior salvage therapy among the commonly used regimens such as DHAP, ICE, IGEV; maintaining dose-intensity is important for optimal responses.
- Functional imaging using FDG-PET scanning after salvage chemotherapy and before ASCT is a critical predictor of outcome; the goal of salvage should be a negative FDG-PET scan.
- Either a second line of salvage or a tandem ASCT may benefit some patients with residual FDG avidity post-salvage.
- RIC-alloSCT may provide a GVL effect and durable responses in some patients with HL relapsing or progressing after ASCT.
- New agents, particularly Brentuximab vedotin, are being incorporated earlier into the treatment of RR-HL, such as those with FDG-avid chemoresistant disease, those progressing through second-line salvage, or those relapsing after an ASCT.

INTRODUCTION

Most patients with Hodgkin lymphoma (HL) are cured by chemotherapy alone with or without additional external beam radiation; however, up to 10% of patients with early-stage favorable HL and up to 30% of patients with early-stage unfavorable or

Disclosure Statement: The author has no conflicts of interest or any interests to declare.
Department of Haematology, Level 2 ICPMR, Westmead Hospital, Darcy Road, Westmead, New South Wales 2145, Australia
E-mail address: mhertzberg10@gmail.com

Hematol Oncol Clin N Am 28 (2014) 123–147
http://dx.doi.org/10.1016/j.hoc.2013.09.001
0889-8588/14/$ – see front matter © 2014 Elsevier Inc. All rights reserved.

hemonc.theclinics.com

advanced stage disease will either fail to respond to first-line therapy or relapse after an initial complete remission (CR). For those who relapse or fail to achieve a CR, standard therapy involves salvage chemotherapy followed by high-dose chemotherapy (HDCT) and autologous stem cell transplantation (ASCT).[1–6] Approximately 40% to 50% of RR-HL patients can be cured with HDCT/ASCT, particularly those with more favorable risk features. In contrast, patients with primary refractory disease and/or adverse risk features at relapse, such as extranodal disease or short response duration, may benefit more from other interventions. These alternative approaches include antibody-drug conjugates and reduced-intensity conditioning allogeneic stem cell transplantation (RIC-alloSCT).

SALVAGE THERAPY AND HDCT/ASCT
Which Prognostic Factors at Progression/Relapse Are Important?

Over the last 20 years, there have been several reports identifying key prognostic factors in patients with relapsed/refractory Hodgkin lymphoma (RR-HL) who have undergone salvage chemotherapy and ASCT (Table 1).

1. The Groupe d'Etude des Lymphomes de l'Adulte developed a 2-factor model that included as adverse features short CR1 duration, and extranodal disease at relapse.[10]
2. The Autologous Blood and Marrow Transplant Registry identified 3 adverse risk factors including Karnofsky performance score less than 90%, abnormal lactate dehydrogenase (LDH) at ASCT, and chemoresistant relapse.[12]
3. Some of the largest studies of prognostic variables have been conducted by the German Hodgkin study group (GHSG).
   a. In their first analysis of 206 patients with primary progressive disease they identified 3 adverse risk factors including ECOGPS greater than 0, age greater than 50 years, and failure to obtain a temporary remission to initial therapy.[11]
   b. In a subsequent study among 422 patients with relapsed HL, they defined a GHSG Clinical Risk Score using 3 adverse prognostic factors for overall survival (OS) including advanced disease stage III/IV, initial response duration of less than 12 months, and anemia (Hb <120 g/L and <105 g/L in men and women).[17] Rates of freedom from second failure at 5 years for patients failing first-line therapy were 45%, 32%, and 18%, for patients with prognostic scores of 0 to 1, 2, and 3, respectively. Hence, this score has been used widely in prospective trials and treatment approaches.
4. From other large studies, consistent adverse prognostic factors have emerged: short initial response duration, usually within 12 months, advanced stage III/IV at relapse, and extranodal disease (see Table 1).[9,10,12,13,17,19–21,26,27]
5. Finally, in a prospective study of ifosfamide, carboplatin, etoposide (ICE) salvage among 85 patients, Moskowitz and colleagues[13] developed a prognostic model of 3 adverse risk factors at relapse, including B symptoms, extranodal disease, and CR duration less than 12 months. The presence of 0 to 1 risk factors was associated with an event-free survival (EFS) of 83%, decreasing to 10% for 3 risk factors.

Which Salvage Regimen?

There are no randomized controlled trials (RCTs) and no consensus as to the most effective salvage regimen for RR-HL. The 2 published RCTs of ASCT (see Table 2) used mini-BCNU, etoposide, cytarabine, melphalan (BEAM) or dexa-BEAM as salvage.[28,29] Although these regimens would still be considered standard, several alternative salvage combinations have been used, reporting overlapping response rates from 60% to 85% (Table 2).[13,15,26,30–42]

Table 1
Prognostic factors for patients with RR-HL

Reference: Author/Year	N	Prognostic Factors
A. RR-HL to 1st Line		
Lohri et al,[7] 1991	80	Stage IV at diagnosis, B symptoms at relapse, 1st response <12 mo
Reece et al,[8] 1994	58	B symptoms, extranodal disease, 1st response <12 mo
Brice et al,[9] 1996	187	1st response <12 mo, stage III/IV at relapse, relapse in prior irradiated field
Brice et al,[10] 1997	260	1st response <12 mo, extranodal relapse
Josting et al,[11] 2000	206	ECOGPS >0, age >50 y, no temporary remission to 1st line
Lazarus et al,[12] 2001	414	Karnofsky PS <90%, abnormal LDH at SCT, chemoresistance to salvage
Moskowitz et al,[13] 2001	65	B symptoms, extranodal disease, response <12 mo
Sureda et al,[14] 2001	494	TTF: chemoresistance at ASCT, $\geq$2 CT lines; OS: ASCT before 1992, $\geq$2 lines of therapy
Ferme et al,[15] 2002	157	"B" symptoms at progression, salvage without ASCT, and chemoresistance to salvage
Bierman et al,[16] 2002	379	IPS factors: serum albumin, anemia, age $\geq$45 y, lymphocytopenia
Josting et al,[17] 2002	422	GHSG Clinical Risk Score: 1st response <12 mo, stage III/IV at relapse, anemia (men <120 g/L, women <105 g/L)
Czyz et al,[18] 2004	341	<PR at ASCT, $\geq$3 prior CT lines
Popat et al,[19] 2004	184	Chemoresistance to salvage, stage III/IV, >2 prior CT lines
Sureda et al,[20] 2005	357	Year of transplant before 1995, CR1 $\leq$12 mo, chemoresistance, and $\geq$1 extranodal site at ASCT
Josting et al,[21] 2010	241	Stage IV (not III), early or multiple relapse, anemia
Balzarotti et al,[22] 2013	330	Refractory to 1st line, age >40 y, bulk, B symptoms
B. Relapse After ASCT		
Martinez et al,[23] 2013	511	Relapse <6 mo after ASCT, stage IV, bulky disease, poor PS, and age $\geq$50 y at relapse
von Tresckow et al,[24] 2013	149	Stage III/IV and B symptoms both present at relapse before ASCT
Arai et al,[25] 2013	756	TTR after ASCT of 0–3 mo, >3–6 mo, >6–12 mo

Abbreviations: CT, chemotherapy; ECOGPS, Eastern Cooperative Oncology Group performance status; IPS, international prognostic score (Hasenclever index); KPS, Karnofsky performance score; LN, lymph node; MOPP, mustine, oncovin, procarbazine, prednisone.

Because most studies incorporate both relapsed and primary refractory HL patients, it is difficult to compare OR and CR rates between regimens. Hematological toxicity is the predominant factor limiting dose intensity, although gastrointestinal (eg, DHAP, Dexa-BEAM) and neurologic (augmented ICE, ifosfamide, gemcitabine, vinorelbine, prednisone) toxicities are also seen. Furthermore, the optimal number of cycles of salvage therapy is not known, although usually 2 to 3 cycles are used, given likely further toxicity and no proven gain in efficacy with additional cycles.

The independent prognostic relevance of dose-density of salvage was also confirmed in the GHSG HDR2 study in relation to progression-free survival (PFS) and OS, thereby supporting the mandatory use of granulocyte colony stimulating factor and in this case the minimal DHAP cycle duration of 14 days.[43]

Table 2
Selected trials of salvage chemotherapy before ASCT

Regimen	Reference: Author/Year	Number Evaluable	ORR (%)	CR (%)	Toxicity
Dexa-BEAM	Schmitz et al,[30] 2002	144	81	27	5.5% toxic deaths
Mini-BEAM	Martin et al,[26] 2001	55	84	51	IV ANC 86%; 2% deaths
MINE	Ferme et al,[15] 2002	83	75	NA	5% toxic deaths (including ASCT)
ICE	Moskowitz et al,[13] 2001	65	88	26	III/IV ANC NR; no toxic deaths
ESHAP	Aparicio et al,[31] 1999	22	73	41	III/IV ANC 59%; 5% toxic deaths
MINE-ESHAP	Fernandez de Larrea et al,[32] 2010	61	79	41	III/IV ANC 46% TCP 40%; 0 toxic deaths
ASHAP	Rodriguez et al,[33] 1999	56	70	34	III/IV ANC 100%; II/III TCP 100%; no toxic deaths
DHAP q2 wk	Josting et al,[34] 2002	102	89	21	IV ANC 43%; IV TCP 48%; no toxic deaths
GDP	Baetz et al,[35] 2003	23	70	17	III/IV ANC/TCP 13%; no toxic deaths
GVD	Bartlett et al,[36] 2007	91	70	19	III/IV ANC 63% TCP 14%; no toxic deaths
IGEV	Santoro et al,[37] 2007	91	81	54	III/IV ANC 28% TCP 20%; no toxic deaths
IVE	Proctor et al,[42] 2003	51	84	60	III/IV ANC 100%; no toxic deaths
DICEP	Shafey et al,[39] 2012	73	86	18	III/IV 1.4% toxic deaths
IVOx	Sibon et al,[40] 2011	34	76	32	III/IV ANC 9%; no toxic deaths
O-ESHAP	Martinez et al,[41] 2012	45	63	49	III/IV ANC 20%; no toxic deaths

Abbreviations: ANC, absolute neutrophil count (neutropenia); ASHAP, doxorubicin, methylprednisolone, cytarabine, cis-platin; Dexa-BEAM, dexamethasone, BCNU, etoposide, cytarabine, melphalan; DHAP, dexamethasone, cytarabine, cis-platin; DICEP, dose-intensified cyclophosphamide, etoposide, cis-platin; ESHAP, etoposide, methylprednisolone, cytarabine, cis-platin; GDP, gemcitabine, dexamethasone, cis-platin; GVD, gemcitabine, vinorelbine, liposomal doxorubicin; IGEV, ifosfamide, gemcitabine, vinorelbine, prednisone; IVE, ifosfamide, etoposide, epirubicin; IVOx, ifosfamide, etoposide, oxaliplatin; MINE: mitoguazone, ifosfamide, vinorelbine, and etoposide; mini-BEAM, BCNU, etoposide, cytarabine, melphalan; NR, not reported; O-ESHAP, ofatumumab, etoposide, methylprednisolone, cytarabine, cis-platin; ORR, overall response rate; TCP, thrombocytopenia.

Why Give HDCT and ASCT?

HDCT/ASCT is considered standard of care for RR-HL patients. The evidence derives from only 2 RCTs comparing HDCT/ASCT conventional chemotherapy. One trial closed prematurely because patients refused randomization and requested ASCT. Although each trial showed no significant improvement in OS, however, PFS was significantly improved with HDCT/ASCT.[28,29]

In a recent systematic review, the Cochrane Collaboration confirmed a nonstatistically significant trend for improved OS for HDCT/ASCT compared with conventional chemotherapy (HR 0.67; 95% CI 0.41–1.07; $P = .1$, 157 patients).[44] However, again there was a statistically significant increase in PFS for HDCT/ASCT (HR 0.55; 95% CI 0.35 to 0.86; $P = .009$, 157 patients).

Are There Differences Between Preparative Regimens for ASCT?

There have been no prospective comparative studies of conditioning regimens for ASCT. At present, there are insufficient data to recommend one conditioning regimen over another. Most studies have used either BEAM or cyclophosphamide, BCNU, VP16 (CBV) conditioning, although more intensive preparative regimens have been used successfully.[45–49]

1. BEAM versus CBV: The Nebraska group recently undertook a retrospective review of 225 RR-HL patients who were alive and disease-free 2 years after ASCT using either BEAM or CBV conditioning.[50] At 5 years, the PFS was 92% for BEAM and 73% for CBV ($P = .002$) and the OS was 95% for BEAM and 87% for CBV ($P = .07$), whereas at 10 years the differences were maintained. They could not exclude the possibility that the superior outcomes seen in the BEAM group were because of better supportive care, use of peripheral blood stem cells, or improvements in salvage therapies before transplantation.[50]
2. Busulphan plus Melphalan: Conditioning with GemBuMel has been shown by Nieto and colleagues[51] to be feasible and effective in a group of 84 patients with RR-HL. Multivariate analyses showed independent adverse effects of a conditioning regimen different from Gem-Bu-Mel (HR for EFS = 2.3, $P = .0008$; HR for OS = 2.7, $P = .0005$). Similarly, Bains and colleagues[52] undertook a retrospective comparison of 60 patients who received novel conditioning with BuMelTt and 40 who received other regimens. At a median follow-up of 4.3 years, the estimated 5-year OS and PFS were superior for patients treated with BuMelTt (73% vs 44%, $P = .05$) and (66% vs 37%, $P = .03$). As a cautionary note, these latter regimens incorporating BuMel are associated with more severe mucositis.

Why Evaluate Response to Salvage Using FDG-PET Pre-ASCT?

In addition to the prognostic factors described above, several studies have shown that functional imaging (FI) (usually positron emission tomography, PET) after salvage chemotherapy and before ASCT is a critical predictor of outcome.[53–60] All these studies report a substantially inferior long-term PFS in patients who are PET-positive (23%–52%) after salvage chemotherapy compared with those who are PET-negative (69%–88%) (**Table 3**). Moreover, in most of these studies, univariate and multivariate analyses indicate that pre-ASCT PET status was the only prognostic factor for PFS/EFS after transplant. Hence, PET scanning after salvage may be a powerful prognostic tool that could be applied to the selection of patients for either or both ASCT, consolidation therapy (eg, tandem ASCT), maintenance agents, or RIC-alloSCT.[58,62,64]

Prospectively, FDG-PET scanning has already been used as part of a response-adapted approach in which patients with 0 to 2 risk factors (B symptoms, extranodal disease, and CR <12 months) who achieve less than a complete metabolic CR (mCR) to initial salvage chemotherapy go on to receive second-line salvage. Moskowitz and colleagues[62] used 2 cycles of ICE in a standard or augmented dose, followed by restaging PET scan. PET-negative patients received an ASCT; PET-positive patients received 4 biweekly doses of a second salvage regimen gemcitabine, vinorelbine, liposomal doxorubicin (see **Table 3**). Patients without evidence of disease progression proceeded to ASCT; those with progressive disease were study failures. At a median follow-up of 51 months, EFS analyzed by both intent to treat and for transplanted

Table 3
Prognostic relevance of FDG-PET scanning postsalvage and pre-ASCT

Reference: Author/Year	Patient No.	PFS PET-ve	PFS PET+ve	P Value	Prognostic Relevance
Jabbour et al,[55] 2007	211	3-y 69% (FI)	3-y 23% (FI)	<.0001	PFS = B symptoms, CR/CRu pre-ASCT, BEAM, FI-pos
		87% (OS)	58% (OS)	<.0001	OS = CR/CRu pre-ASCT, IFRT initially, and BEAM
Moskowitz et al,[53] 2010	153	5-y 75% (FI)	5-y 31% (FI)	<.0001	OS and PFS: FI alone
Moskowitz et al,[54] 2010	105	4-y 77% (FI)	4-y 33% (FI)	.00004	FI eliminated difference between 3 prognostic groups
Mocikova et al,[61] 2011	76	2-y 72.7% 90.3% (OS)	2-y 36.2% 61.4% (OS)	.01 .009	PET = ns in multivariate
Smeltzer et al,[56] 2011	46	3-y 82%	3-y 41%	.02	PET for EFS (HR 3.2, P = .03)
Sucak et al,[57] 2011	43	3-y 70.6%	3-y 37.6%	.008	PFS: PET-pos pre- and post-ASCT. OS: PET-pos post-ASCT only
Devillier et al,[58] 2012	111	5-y 79%	5-y 23%	<.001	PFS: PET (HR: 5.26) and tandem ASCT (HR: 0.39) but not the SFGM 3 risk factors
		90% (OS)	55% (OS)	.001	OS: PET only (HR, 4.03)
Moskowitz et al,[62] 2012	97	4-y 80%	4-y 28.6%	<.001	After 1 or 2 salvage regimens (ICE, GVD)
Akhtar et al,[63] 2013	141	NR	NR	.011 (OS)	Disease-related death: postsalvage PET (P = .011); HR: 3.4 (1.3–8.9). Disease-specific event: postsalvage PET (P = .001); HR: 3.3 (1.7–6.7)
Nassi et al,[60] 2013	54	5-y 88%	5-y 42%	.0001	PPV = 58% and NPV = 88%
Bramanti et al,[59] 2013	67	3-y 84% 94% (OS)	3-y 52% 60% (OS)	.008 .002	PET2 and PET4 for PFS (P = .01)

Abbreviations: GVD, gemcitabine, vinorelbine, liposomal doxorubicin; SFGM, Société Française de Greffe de Moelle; TTP, time to progression.

patients was 70% and 79%, respectively. Patients transplanted with negative pre-ASCT PET (after 1 or 2 salvage regimens) had an EFS of greater than 80% versus 28.6% for PET-positive patients (P<.001). Notably, there was no difference in EFS and OS between relapsed and refractory patients. These data argue that the goal of salvage in patients with RR-HL should be a negative FDG-PET scan before ASCT.

Can Results of ASCT Be Improved by Sequential HDCT or Tandem ASCT?

Other attempts to intensify the salvage therapy have included additional sequential HDCT (SHDCT), or tandem ASCT.

SHDCT

There has been one RCT, the HDR2 study, evaluating the effect of SHDCT before ASCT in 284 relapsed HL patients.[21] All patients received 2 cycles of DHAP, followed either directly by ASCT with BEAM, or first by sequential cyclophosphamide, methotrexate, and etoposide before BEAM. Both the final trial analysis and the analysis undertaken by the Cochrane Collaboration found no difference between treatment arms for OS (HR 0.93; P = .86, 3-year OS: 80% SHDCT vs 87% HDCT) or PFS (HR 0.87; P = .505).[44] There was also no benefit for SHDCT for those patients in early relapse (3–12 months) following initial induction therapy.

Tandem ASCT

Five phase II studies addressed the role of tandem ASCT in RR-HL (**Table 4**).[65,67–69] The largest of these trials, the H96 study, evaluated a risk-adapted salvage treatment with either single or tandem ASCT for 245 patients.[68] Poor-risk patients (n = 150) had primary refractory HL (n = 77) or unfavorable relapse ($\geq$2 risk factors: time to relapse <12 months, stage III/IV, and relapse within previously irradiated sites, n = 73) and were eligible for tandem ASCT. Intermediate-risk patients (n = 95) had one risk factor at first relapse and were eligible for a single ASCT. The 45% 5-year OS in patients with first-line chemotherapy-resistant disease who completed tandem

Table 4				
Tandem autoSCT studies				
Reference: Author/Year	N	Preparative Regimen	FFP	OS
Brice et al,[65] 1999	42 39 (asct-1) 32 (asct-2)	IVA75 salvage: 1. CBV + Mitox 2. AraC + Mel + TBI or Bu	2-y 65% (itt) 2-y 74% (asct-2)	2-y 65% (itt) 2-y 74% (asct-2)
Castagna et al,[66] 2007	32 29 (asct-1) 27 (asct-2)	IGEV salvage: 1. Mel 200 2. BEAM	3-y 63% (itt)	3-y 79% (itt)
Fung et al,[67] 2007	46 44 (asct-1) 41 (asct-2)	Cy/Et or other salvage: 1. Mel 150 2. Cy + Et + BCNU or TBI	5-y 49% (itt) 5-y 49% (asct-2)	5-y 54% (itt) 5-y 57% (asct-2)
Morschhauser et al,[68] 2008	150 (bad risk) 137 (asct-1) 118 (asct-2)	IVA75 or MINE salvage: 1. CBV-Mx or BEAM 2. TAM or BAM	5-y 41%–52% (itt) 5-y 36%–64% (asct-2)	5-y 53%–61% (itt) 5-y 45%–75% (asct-2)
Dean et al,[69] 2012	42 37 (asct-1) 37 (asct-2)	Mixed salvage: 1. Mel 150 2. CBV or BuCyEt	Med = 15.5 mo (asct-2) vs = 26.3 mo in controls	Med = 54.9 mo (asct-2) vs = 73.1 mo in controls

Abbreviations: Ara-C, cytarabine; asct-1, asct-2, autologous stem cell transplant 1st, 2nd; BAM, busulfan, cytarabine, and melphalan; Bu, Busulphan; Cy, cyclophosphamide; Et, etoposide; FFP, freedom from progression; itt, intention to treat; IVA, ifosfamide, etoposide, doxorubicin; Mel, Melphalan; Mx, mitoxantrone; TAM, total-body irradiation, cytarabine, and melphalan; TBI, total body irradiation; Thio, thiotepa.

transplant compares favorably with previously reported 5-year OS rates of 30%. At a recent 10-year follow-up, freedom from treatment failure and OS were 64% and 70%, respectively, for the intermediate-risk group (single ASCT), and 40% and 47%, respectively, for the poor-risk group (tandem ASCT).[70]

In a recent retrospective analysis, Devillier and colleagues[58] described 111 patients who were assigned to either a single or tandem ASCT depending on a combination of the 3 SFGM adverse prognostic factors at relapse and PET responsiveness to salvage. They showed that PET status before ASCT was a much stronger predictor of outcomes than classical risk factors at relapse, and that tandem ASCT could be superior to single ASCT (5-year PFS of 74% vs 48%, respectively, $P = .002$). Furthermore, in the PET-positive group, tandem ASCT improved the 5-year PFS from 0% in the single ASCT to 43% ($P = .034$).

Taken together, these studies suggest that a tandem ASCT may represent an effective option for a substantial subset of poor risk RR-HL patients.

Can Results of ASCT Be Improved by Incorporating Novel Agents?

Recent strategies designed to improve the results of HDCT/ASCT have added novel agents such as Brentuximab vedotin (BV) either to the salvage regimen (ESHAP, DHAP) or as post-ASCT maintenance, particularly in those patients considered at high risk of relapse.

1. In a current phase III trial (AETHERA) those deemed at high risk of relapse (primary refractory, relapsed/progressive HL <12 months from frontline therapy, or extranodal involvement at relapse) are randomized to placebo or maintenance BV (www.ClinicalTrials.gov No. NCT01100502).
2. An important question is whether BV could replace ICE or DHAP salvage.[71] With that in mind, investigators at MSKCC are evaluating single-agent BV as initial pre-ASCT salvage (www.ClinicalTrials.gov No. NCT01508312). PET-negative patients after 2 BV cycles proceed to ASCT; FDG-avid patients receive 2 cycles of augmented dose ICE followed by ASCT.
3. In addition, a phase II study in patients with primary refractory or progressive HL after standard frontline therapy is evaluating salvage with single-agent BV (maximum 4 cycles) before ASCT (www.ClinicalTrials.gov No. NCT01393717).

What is the Prognosis for Patients Who Relapse Post-ASCT?

Among chemosensitive patients with relapsed HL, 40% to 50% will fail to respond to salvage chemotherapy and HDCT/ASCT; among patients refractory to first-line therapy, up to 60% to 75% will fail to respond.[20]

1. From a large retrospective analysis of the EBMT-GITMO databases 511 patients were identified who relapsed after ASCT (see **Table 1**).[23] Treatment included conventional chemotherapy and/or radiation in 294 (64%), a second ASCT in 35 (8%), and an alloSCT in 133 (29%). Independent risk factors for OS were early relapse less than 6 months after ASCT, stage IV, bulk, poor ECOGPS, and age ≥50 years. At 5 years, OS ranged from 62% for those with no risk factors to 12% for those with ≥2 risk factors.
2. The GHSG identified 149 patients who relapsed or progressed after ASCT.[24] For the entire group, the median survival was less than 2 years with 20% survival at 5 years. For those with the 0, 1, and 2 risk factors (stage III/IV and B symptoms before ASCT), 5-year OS was 41%, 27%, and 8%, respectively (see **Table 1**).
3. OS strongly correlates with the time to relapse after ASCT; for patients who relapse within 6 months of ASCT, median survival is 1.5 years.[72] These adverse outcomes

were again highlighted in a recent international collaborative analysis of 756 patients, which showed the median OS and PFS after ASCT failure was 2.4 years and 1.3 years.[25] The data confirmed time to relapse after ASCT as a prognostic factor, with median PPS of 0.98 versus 2.26 years for relapses less than 12 months or greater than 12 months, respectively.

These correlates of prognostic factors and survival outcomes help to identify post-ASCT relapsing patients as a reference group for whom novel strategies can be assessed.[73–75]

DO WE NEED RIC-ALLOSCT FOR RR-HL?

The standard of care for patients whose disease progresses or relapses following an autoSCT has not been fully established and has led to exploration of allogeneic SCT, which combines the antitumor effect of chemotherapy with the potential advantage of a graft-versus-lymphoma (GVL) effect mediated by donor T cells and natural killer cells.

There have been no randomized comparisons between a second ASCT and an alloSCT. Numerous retrospective comparisons have been performed. Notwithstanding the caveats of such analyses including the patient heterogeneity, and the use of both myeloablative conditioning (MAC) and RIC, these studies do suggest the presence of a long-term survival benefit for allo-SCT in a subset of patients with high-risk RR-HL.[76–82]

What About Myeloablative Allogeneic SCT?

MAC derives its benefit from a combination of the intensive preparative regimen and the putative GVL effect. However, MAC is associated with high rates of nonrelapse mortality (NRM) ranging from 39% to 61%.[76–82] The high NRM is likely a result of the cumulative toxicity of previous combined modality treatments, intensive salvage chemotherapy, selection of high-risk patients with advanced disease, and the immunodeficiency seen commonly in HL that predisposes patients to infectious complications.

What Is the Advantage of RIC-alloSCT Compared to MAC?

Direct comparisons of MAC and RIC regimens are difficult because patients are often selected for the latter because of prior extensive therapy or comorbidities. Nevertheless, in the largest series comparing MAC with RIC, Sureda and colleagues[82] showed that RIC significantly decreases NRM even in patients with poor prognostic features at the time of allograft with a 3-year NRM of 24% for RIC versus 48% for MAC. In that study, the improved NRM associated with RIC-alloSCT was offset substantially by the increase in disease progression/relapse of 58% versus 32% for RIC and MAC, respectively. In other studies, reduced NRM rates of 8% to 24% have translated into a better OS and a trend toward better PFS for patients treated with the RIC regimens (**Table 5**).

Which Retrospective Studies of RIC-AlloSCT Are Informative?

There have been several retrospective reports of RIC-alloSCT in RR-HL (see **Table 5**).[82–84,86,89–93,95–100,108,109] These reports have included the following few key studies:

1. The MDACC reported the data of RIC-alloSCT using Flu/Mel ± anti-thymocyte globulin (ATG) in 58 HL patients of whom 48% were chemorefractory and 29%

Table 5
RIC-allo SCT studies in RR-HL

Reference: Author/Year	Conditioning	N	Prior ASCT (%)	Prior Regimens (Median)	NRM (%)	CIR (%)	PFS (%)	OS (%)
Robinson et al,[83] 2002	FluMel (±AI) or FluBu or FluCy	52	69	3	2-y 17.3	2-y 45.8	2-y 42	2-y 56.3
Alvarez et al,[84] 2006	FluMel	40	73	2	1-y 25	2-y 43	2-y 32	2-y 48
Peggs et al,[85] 2005	FluMel + AI	41	90	5	2-y 16.3	4-y 43	4-y 39	4-y 55.7
Baron et al,[86] 2006	FluTBI-2 Gy	35	92	NR	3-y 32	3-y 60–70	3-y 8	3-y 35
Majhail et al,[87] 2006	FluTBI-2 Gy ± Cy	9 UCB 12 RD	78 58	2	6 mo 22 25	NR	2-y 25 20	2-y 51 48
Peggs et al,[85,88] 2005, 2007 Alvarez et al,[84] 2006	FluMel + AI	31	87	5	2-y 7	3-y 54	4-y 39	4-y 62
	FluMel + MTX	36	72	2	29	44	25	39
Anderlini et al,[89,90] 2005, 2008	FluMel ± ATG	58	83	5	2-y 15	2-y 55	2-y 32	2-y 64
Armand et al,[91] 2008	FluBu	36	94	4	3-y 15	3-y 63	3-y 22	3-y 56
Burroughs et al,[92] 2008	FluTBI-2 Gy ± Cy (haplo)	90 Sib 38 UD 24 Haplo 28	92	5	2-y 21 8 9	2-y 56 63 40	2-y 23 29 51	2-y 53 58 58
Sureda et al,[82] 2008	RIC	89	62	3	3-y 24	5-y 58	5-y 18	5-y 28
	MAC	79	41	3	3-y 48	5-y 32	5-y 20	5-y 22
Thomson et al,[93] 2008	FluMel + Alem	38	100	3	5-y 19	5-y 55	5-y 34	5-y 51

Study	Conditioning	N						
Castagna et al,[94] 2009	FluCy or FluMelTBI-2 Gy	26	100	2	1-y 8	2-y 50	2-y 47	2-y 71
Devetten et al,[95] 2009	FluMel, FluBu, Flu + TBI-2Gy-Cy	143	89	3	2-y 33	2-y 47	2-y 20	2-y 37
Robinson et al,[96] 2009	FluMel, FluBu or FluCy	285	80	4	3-y 21.1	5-y 58.7	3-y 25	3-y 29
Kuruvilla et al,[97] 2010	FluCy, FluBu or FluMel	29	97	3	17	69	3-y 19	3-y 42
Sarina et al,[98] 2010	FluCy ± Tt or FluMel	104	100	NR	2-y 12.7	2-y 54	2-y 31	2-y 57
Chen et al,[99] 2011	FluMel	24	83	5	2-y 13	2-y 63	2-y 27	2-y 60
Johansson et al,[100] 2011	FluMel, FluBu or FluCy	23	87	5	1-y 22	3-y 57	3-y 27	3-y 59
Anderlini et al,[101] 2012	GemFluMel ± ATG	15	47	4	18 mo 13	NR	18 mo 49	18 mo 87
Sobol et al,[102] 2012	BEAM ± ATG	31	NR	5	1-y 13	NR	7-y 36	7-y 42
Sureda et al,[103] 2012	FluMel ± ATG	92	86	2	4-y 19	4-y 59	4-y 24	4-y 43
Chen et al,[104,105] 2012, 2013	BV then RIC-alloSCT	18	94	4	2-y 13.8	2-y 29.4	2-y 57.5	2-y 79
Marcais et al,[106] 2013	FluBu, FluMel or FluTBI-2 Gy ± ATG	191	92	>2	3-y 16	3-y 46	3-y 39	3-y 63
Bacigalupo et al,[107] 2013	Haplo FluCyTBI-2 Gy	26	100	NR	2-y 4	2-y 31	2-y 63	3-y 77
Thomson et al,[64] 2013	BEAM-Al	25	0	3	3-y 8	3-y 24	3-y 68	3-y 88

Abbreviations: Al, alemtuzumab; Bu, busulphan; Cy, cyclophosphamide; Mel, melphalan; NR, not reported; RIC, reduced intensity conditioning; TBI, total body irradiation, usually at 2 Gy; Tt, thiotepa; UCB, unrelated cord blood.

had no prior ASCT.[89,90] At 2 years, NRM was 15%, whereas PFS and OS were 32% and 64%, respectively, with no outcome difference between unrelated donor (UD) and related donor (RD) transplants.

2. The EBMT described the largest series of HL patients treated with RIC-alloSCT.[96] This study included 285 heavily pretreated HL patients of whom 17% were in CR, 43% had chemosensitive disease, and 40% had chemoresistance or untested relapse. Three-year NRM was 21.1%, whereas 3-year PFS was 25%, which was significantly worse for those with chemoresistant disease ($P<.001$).

3. In the largest retrospective comparison of RIC-alloSCT versus conventional treatment after a failed ASCT, the GITMO reported results only for patients with available antigen typing immediately after a failed ASCT.[98] Of 185 patients, 122 found a matched RD (55%), UD (32%), or a haploidentical (haplo) donor (13%), whereas 63 patients did not find any donor. Two-year PFS and OS were better in the donor group (39.3% vs 14.2%, and 66% vs 42%, respectively, $P<.001$) with a median follow-up of 48 months. In multivariate analysis, having a donor was significantly better for PFS and OS ($P<.001$) as was time from autoSCT to relapse of less than 12 months versus greater than 12 months ($P = .023$); patients allografted in CR showed a better PFS and OS. In both donor and no donor groups the most common cause of treatment failure was disease progression. As seen elsewhere, the NRM did not differ significantly between the donor and no donor groups.[82,85,96]

4. The SFGM-TC (Société Française de Greffe de Moelle et de Thérapie Cellulaire) has reported a large study of RIC-alloSCT in RR-HL. Between 1998 and 2008, 191 patients underwent RIC-alloSCT conditioned with FluBu, FluMel, or FluTBI-2 Gy, together with ATG in 43%.[106] Ninety-two percent (171) of the patients had undergone previous ASCT and 29% had chemoresistant disease at the time of RIC-alloSCT. At a median follow-up of 36 months, the estimated 3-year OS, PFS, cumulative incidence of relapse (CIR), and NRM were 63%, 39%, 46%, and 16%, respectively. Notably, there was no difference in outcome between patients in CR and in PR at the time of SCT for OS (70% vs 74%) and PFS (51% vs 42%). However, compared with those in CR, patients with chemoresistant disease had a shorter OS (39% at 3 years $P = .0003$) and PFS (18% at 3 years $P = .001$). These results suggested that even for patients in PR, RIC-alloSCT should be offered, whereas it was difficult to justify RIC-alloSCT alone for patients with chemoresistant disease given the dismal outcomes in this setting.

From a practical viewpoint, these findings provide support for the feasibility and efficacy of RIC-alloSCT in association with lower rates of NRM than MAC in heavily pretreated HL patients.

Are There Prospective Studies of RIC-alloSCT?

No prospective randomized studies between RIC-alloSCT and salvage chemoradiotherapy have been conducted in HL patients relapsing after an ASCT. Only one retrospective study by Thomson and colleagues[93] has been published on this topic, showing the superiority of RIC-alloSCT over conventional treatment (see **Table 5**). Nevertheless, that study had some limitations including that less than 40 patients were included in each arm, and that only those responding to salvage therapy and surviving more than 12 months were included in the control group.

The GEL/TAMO group reported results of a large prospective phase II study of 92 RR-HL patients and a matched RD or UD of whom 86% had undergone a prior ASCT.[103] Fourteen patients showed refractory disease and died of progressive HL with a median OS of 10 months (range, 6–17). Seventy-eight patients proceeded to

RIC-alloSCT including 23 UD transplants; 50 patients were allografted in CR or PR and 28 in stable disease. The conditioning regimen consisted of FluMel, plus ATG for UD transplants. For the allografted population the 4-year NRM, CIR, PFS, and OS were 19%, 59%, 24%, and 43%, respectively. Chronic GVHD was associated with a lower incidence of relapse, whereas patients allografted in CR had a significantly better outcome.

Overall, the favorable results from these retrospective and prospective studies of RIC-alloSCT, particularly the low NRM of 10% at 1 year, provide strong support for this modality among post-ASCT relapsing patients. Nevertheless, although the RIC-alloSCT approach significantly reduced NRM, the high relapse rate represents the major challenge in this setting.

What Prognostic Factors Before RIC-alloSCT Are Important?

In HL, it is well established that chemorefractory patients experience a short survival, because the GVL effect cannot overcome the aggressive clinical course of the disease.[82–84,106] Conversely, there are conflicting data as to whether the CR or PR status at transplantation affects outcome. Some studies showed that PR and chemorefractory HL patients experienced the same outcome, suggesting that only CR before RIC-alloSCT should be pursued to allow the immune-mediated effect to be exerted in the long term.[85,90,96] In addition, there are differences in PFS and OS for CR patients versus PR patients, supporting the notion that pretransplantation CR status is crucial to improve the outcome.[98,106] In contrast, the SGFM study showed no difference in outcomes between patients in CR or PR before RIC-alloSCT.[106]

The only study examining the effect of FDG-PET scanning before RIC-alloSCT was a retrospective analysis of 46 patients with RR-HL of whom 91% had undergone a prior ASCT. They confirmed that a negative pre-alloSCT PET scan significantly predicted the risk of PFS (3-year 72% vs 30%, $P = .027$) and OS (3-year 82% vs 28%, $P = .006$) and was independent of GVHD.[110] The major caveat to this interpretation was that different donor types were included and this alone impacted on OS. Nevertheless, it may suggest the need for additional bridging therapy to improve the response before RIC-alloSCT.

Taking these studies together, chemosensitivity and CR status (ideally determined by FDG-PET) at the time of RIC-alloSCT represent the most important factors in improving outcomes, suggesting that pretransplant disease control is one of the major determinants of long-term survival.[111]

Does Donor Type Matter?

For allografted patients the donor type does not seem to effect toxicity or survival.

1. The CIBMTR described the outcome of the largest group of UD alloSCT recipients, showing a 2-year PFS and OS of 20% and 37%, respectively, similar to the ones obtained with sibling donors.[95]
2. The EBMT report on RIC-alloSCT in HL did not identify the alternative donor as a risk factor for OS.[96]
3. The Seattle group compared the results of nonmyeloablative alloSCT with RD, UD, or haplo donors, and unexpectedly, haplo recipients displayed the most favorable outcome, although different conditioning regimens and the limited number of patients could have affected the analysis, as highlighted by the authors.[92]
4. The GITMO retrospective study also showed no difference in toxicity or survival between either matched RD or UD transplants.[98]

5. In a systematic review of UD and alternative donor allogeneic SCT, Messer and colleagues[112] identified a total of 13 reports, including 4 direct comparisons of UD and RD transplants, and 3 registry analyses. Results of rates of NRM, GVHD, OS, and PFS showed no consistent tendency in favor of a donor type. For unrelated cord blood, one direct comparative study[87] and 2 noncomparative studies confirmed similar favorable results, whereas one study comparing haplo with RD transplants indicated a benefit in PFS for the haplo group.[112] Another recent report of 26 haplo donor RIC-alloSCT transplants showed encouraging 2-year rates of NRM, CIR, PFS, and OS of 4%, 31%, 63% and 77%, respectively.[107]

Overall, there seems to be no fundamental disadvantage of UD or alternative donor transplants compared with RD transplants for advanced HL.

Are Differences Between RIC-alloSCT Preparative Regimens Relevant?

The ideal conditioning regimen for HL patients undergoing an RIC-alloSCT is not known. A wide diversity of preparative regimens has been used that ranges from truly nonmyeloablative with fludarabine (Flu) and total body irradiation, 2 Gy to more intensive regimens incorporating Mel 140 mg/m^2, Bu up to 6.4 mg/kg, or Cy up to 100 mg/kg (see **Table 5**). The combination of Flu plus Mel-140 has been shown to be effective and safe for most patients with HL.[85,90,103]

As in vivo T-cell depletion, alemtuzumab and ATG have been added to conditioning regimens such as FluMel.[106,113] In a comparative analysis of GVHD prophylaxis of cyclosporin with either alemtuzumab or methotrexate the former resulted in a lower incidence of GVHD, and a lower NRM without a decrease in OS. However, such an approach carries the need for more frequent donor lymphocyte infusions for mixed chimerism or persistent disease.[88] Other studies have used BEAM ± alemtuzumab or GemFluMel each with encouraging results.[64,102]

Is There Evidence For a GVL Effect?

Existence of a GVL effect is also still debated because relapse rates are still high in most studies ranging between 30% and 70% (see **Table 5**). The evidence for a GVL effect derives largely from the fact that (1) relapse rates are lower after allografting compared with ASCT, (2) chronic GVHD is associated with a lower relapse rate, and (3) DLIs can also result in remission and long-term PFS. Several studies have confirmed that relapse rates are lower in those developing GVHD after transplantation.[81,82,84,85,90,92,96,98,106]

Furthermore, the 2 large EBMT analyses showed that chronic GVHD was associated with a lower incidence of relapse; however, these results did not translate into better PFS and OS, mainly due to an increased NRM.[82,96] In these studies, the effect of GVHD on outcome was assessed by a landmark analysis approach and not as a time-dependent variable. When the latter statistical approach was applied to the above SFGM study, patients experiencing extensive chronic GVHD had a lower risk of relapse with an HR of 0.40 ($P = .039$).[106] In the Italian study, patients with chronic GVHD experienced a better OS and PFS ($P<.001$ and $P = .024$, respectively) compared with those without.[98] Taken together, these studies support a likely GVL effect in a substantial subset of RR-HL patients.

Are Donor Lymphocyte Infusions Effective?

The use of DLI in the management of recurrent disease is debated. Several studies have demonstrated a GVL effect from DLI and response rates of 30% to 50% have been reported.[88,113–115]

1. Peggs and colleagues[85] were the first to describe the correlation between clinical response and GVHD occurrence after DLI in patients receiving a T-cell-depleted RIC alloSCT. In a subsequent report the same group provided the outcomes of 76 consecutive patients with multiple relapses or refractory HL who underwent RIC-alloSCT, of whom 45 received DLIs, 22 for mixed chimerism and 24 for relapse (although 10 of these also received salvage therapy).[113] The overall response rate was 79% (including a CR in 30%), and with a favorable duration of response in most cases. In this cohort, in vivo alemtuzumab was used in the conditioning regimen, whereas relapse was lower among those receiving DLIs for mixed chimerism than those who remained relapse-free but with full-donor chimerism. It is postulated that in both contexts, alemtuzumab may impact on the tumor microenvironment providing a better setting for the effect of subsequent DLIs.[116]
2. The MDACC reported 27 patients with RR-HL who received DLIs after an RIC-alloSCT.[114] The rate of CR/PR was 37% and responses were always associated with the development of GVHD, providing support for the GVL effect. However, responses were not always durable such that the actuarial estimated overall survival at 4 years for the group was 20%. Similarly, in the SFGM study, among the 30 evaluable patients, the response rate to DLI was 27%.[106]

Can We Incorporate Alternative Strategies Into the RIC-alloSCT Approach?

PET-adapted approaches

One alternative approach has been to move the allogeneic procedure further up in the treatment strategy of RR-HL patients and to use early PET scanning to select adverse risk patients.

The UK group used a PET-adapted approach in which patients who achieved less than a complete mCR to salvage and had at least stable disease underwent an RIC-alloSCT if they had a matched SD or 8 to 10/10 HLA-matched UD, while those with a mCR proceeded to ASCT.[64] Among 61 RR-HL patients, 28 underwent an ASCT, whereas 25 proceeded to RIC-alloSCT using BEAM-alemtuzumab conditioning in 24 of 25. Of the 25, 20 (80%) were primary resistant, 4 (16%) relapsed at less than 12 months, and 14 (56%) had extranodal disease at relapse, in addition to being PET-positive after salvage. Three-year PFS and OS in the allograft group was 68% and 88%, respectively, with a CIR of 25%. Notably, RIC-alloSCT patients received intensive ASCT-like conditioning with BEAM, and the PET-conversion rate varied. Nevertheless, this strategy is encouraging and must be further validated.

Novel agents

From the accumulated studies described above, there is evidence to suggest that RIC-alloSCT alone may not be sufficient to control several cases of RR-HL. Because chemosensitivity and remission status are critical for achieving favorable outcomes following RIC-alloSCT, current strategies are being designed to achieve a CR by using novel agents such as BV early on, and, if a remission is achieved to consolidate with RIC-alloSCT.[105,117] Accordingly, Chen and colleagues[104] showed that RIC-alloSCT after BV is safe in heavily pretreated relapsed HL patients. Among a cohort of 54 patients treated with BV, 18 of 36 transplant-eligible patients elected for RIC-alloSCT. Two-year rates of PFS and OS were 57.5% and 79%, respectively; the 2-year CIR and NRM were 29.4% and 13.8%, whereas rates of acute GVHD and cGVHD were 67% and 50%, respectively.

A particularly poor risk group of patients includes those who are refractory to, or relapse early (<3 months) after, BEACOPP-escalated chemotherapy induction.[21,118] It is tantalizing to suggest that this cohort in particular could be most readily salvaged early with BV, followed by RIC-alloSCT or an ASCT and RIC-alloSCT in a tandem procedure.

Finally, the GVL effect may also be enhanced using BV salvage ± DLI after a relapse post-RIC-alloSCT.[119,120] In one study, 25 patients relapsing after RIC-alloSCT were treated with BV with an overall response rate of 50% and a CR of 38% and a PFS of 7.8 months.[119] Perhaps BV can contribute to some resetting of the immune system in enhancing a GVL effect.

A TREATMENT ALGORITHM FOR RR-HL

One pragmatic approach to the treatment of RR-HL is outlined in **Fig. 1**. RR-HL patients can receive 2 to 3 cycles of a salvage regimen, such as DHAP, ICE, or ifosfamide, gemcitabine, vinorelbine, prednisone, and then undergo a restaging FDG-PET scan. Chemosensitive patients, confirmed by the presence of an mCR or nodal near mCR, can proceed to HDCT/ASCT plus RT to any nodal FDG-avid sites. Those patients who remain PET-positive to first-line salvage can either undergo a tandem ASCT, or receive a second-line salvage regimen such as gemcitabine, vinorelbine, liposomal doxorubicin followed by an ASCT in PET responders. In the circumstance

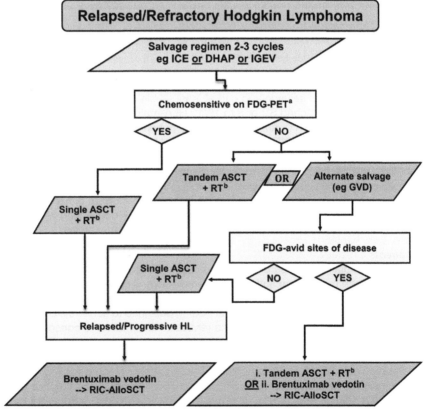

Fig. 1. A treatment algorithm for RR-HL. [a] Chemosensitive = complete or near complete metabolic response (eg, Deauville score ≤4). [b] RT to a residual nodal site of ≥1.5 cm. DHAP, dexamethasone, high-dose cytarabine, cisplatin; GVD, gemcitabine, vinorelbine, liposomal doxorubicin; IGEV, ifosfamide, gemcitabine, vinorelbine.

of progression or PET-positivity after second salvage the evidence is sparse such that no strong evidence-based treatment guideline can be given. Nevertheless, those who display persistent FDG-avidity after second-line salvage can proceed to either tandem ASCT + RT or BV salvage followed by RIC-alloSCT. Similarly, patients who progress through second-line salvage, or those who relapse after ASCT, would be eligible for BV as a bridge to a RIC-alloSCT.

REFERENCES

1. Kuruvilla J, Keating A, Crump M. How I treat relapsed and refractory Hodgkin lymphoma. Blood 2011;117(16):4208–17.
2. Sureda A, Pereira MI, Dreger P, et al. The role of hematopoietic stem cell transplantation in the treatment of relapsed/refractory Hodgkin's lymphoma. Curr Opin Oncol 2012;24(6):727–32.
3. Ramchandren R. Advances in the treatment of relapsed or refractory Hodgkin's lymphoma. Oncologist 2012;17(3):367–76.
4. Mendler JH, Friedberg JW. Salvage therapy in Hodgkin's lymphoma. Oncologist 2009;14(4):425–32.
5. Carella AM. Role of hematopoietic stem cell transplantation in relapsed/refractory Hodgkin lymphoma. Mediterr J Hematol Infect Dis 2012;4(1):e2012059.
6. Holmberg L, Maloney DG. The role of autologous and allogeneic hematopoietic stem cell transplantation for Hodgkin lymphoma. J Natl Compr Canc Netw 2011; 9(9):1060–71.
7. Lohri A, Barnett M, Fairey RN, et al. Outcome of treatment of first relapse of Hodgkin's disease after primary chemotherapy: identification of risk factors from the British Columbia experience 1970 to 1988. Blood 1991;77(10):2292–8.
8. Reece DE, Connors JM, Spinelli JJ, et al. Intensive therapy with cyclophosphamide, carmustine, etoposide +/- cisplatin, and autologous bone marrow transplantation for Hodgkin's disease in first relapse after combination chemotherapy. Blood 1994;83(5):1193–9.
9. Brice P, Bastion Y, Divine M, et al. Analysis of prognostic factors after the first relapse of Hodgkin's disease in 187 patients. Cancer 1996;78(6):1293–9.
10. Brice P, Bouabdallah R, Moreau P, et al. Prognostic factors for survival after high-dose therapy and autologous stem cell transplantation for patients with relapsing Hodgkin's disease: analysis of 280 patients from the French registry. Societe Francaise de Greffe de Moelle. Bone Marrow Transplant 1997;20(1):21–6.
11. Josting A, Rueffer U, Franklin J, et al. Prognostic factors and treatment outcome in primary progressive Hodgkin lymphoma: a report from the German Hodgkin Lymphoma Study Group. Blood 2000;96(4):1280–6.
12. Lazarus HM, Loberiza FR Jr, Zhang MJ, et al. Autotransplants for Hodgkin's disease in first relapse or second remission: a report from the autologous blood and marrow transplant registry (ABMTR). Bone Marrow Transplant 2001;27(4): 387–96.
13. Moskowitz CH, Nimer SD, Zelenetz AD, et al. A 2-step comprehensive high-dose chemoradiotherapy second-line program for relapsed and refractory Hodgkin disease: analysis by intent to treat and development of a prognostic model. Blood 2001;97(3):616–23.
14. Sureda A, Arranz R, Iriondo A, et al. Autologous stem-cell transplantation for Hodgkin's disease: results and prognostic factors in 494 patients from the Grupo Espanol de Linfomas/Transplante Autologo de Medula Osea Spanish Cooperative Group. J Clin Oncol 2001;19(5):1395–404.

15. Ferme C, Mounier N, Divine M, et al. Intensive salvage therapy with high-dose chemotherapy for patients with advanced Hodgkin's disease in relapse or failure after initial chemotherapy: results of the Groupe d'Etudes des Lymphomes de l'Adulte H89 Trial. J Clin Oncol 2002;20(2):467–75.
16. Bierman PJ, Lynch JC, Bociek RG, et al. The international prognostic factors project score for advanced Hodgkin's disease is useful for predicting outcome of autologous hematopoietic stem cell transplantation. Ann Oncol 2002;13(9): 1370–7.
17. Josting A, Franklin J, May M, et al. New prognostic score based on treatment outcome of patients with relapsed Hodgkin's lymphoma registered in the database of the German Hodgkin's lymphoma study group. J Clin Oncol 2002;20(1): 221–30.
18. Czyz J, Dziadziuszko R, Knopinska-Postuszuy W, et al. Outcome and prognostic factors in advanced Hodgkin's disease treated with high-dose chemotherapy and autologous stem cell transplantation: a study of 341 patients. Ann Oncol 2004;15(8):1222–30.
19. Popat U, Hosing C, Saliba RM, et al. Prognostic factors for disease progression after high-dose chemotherapy and autologous hematopoietic stem cell transplantation for recurrent or refractory Hodgkin's lymphoma. Bone Marrow Transplant 2004;33(10):1015–23.
20. Sureda A, Constans M, Iriondo A, et al. Prognostic factors affecting long-term outcome after stem cell transplantation in Hodgkin's lymphoma autografted after a first relapse. Ann Oncol 2005;16(4):625–33.
21. Josting A, Muller H, Borchmann P, et al. Dose intensity of chemotherapy in patients with relapsed Hodgkin's lymphoma. J Clin Oncol 2010;28(34): 5074–80.
22. Balzarotti M, Anastasia A, Ziloli VR, et al. Prognostic factors in patients (PTS) with relapsed/refractory (R/R) Hodgkin's lymphoma (HL) treated with IGEV and autologous stem cell transplantation (ASCT): a Italiana linfomi (fil). Hematol Oncol 2013;31:96–150.
23. Martinez C, Canals C, Sarina B, et al. Identification of prognostic factors predicting outcome in Hodgkin's lymphoma patients relapsing after autologous stem cell transplantation. Ann Oncol 2013;24(9):2430–4.
24. von Tresckow B, Muller H, Eichenauer DA, et al. Outcome and risk factors of Hodgkin lymphoma patients with relapse or progression after autologous stem cell transplant: a report from the German Hodgkin study group (GHSG). Haematologica 2013;98(S1):220.
25. Arai S, Fanale M, Devos S, et al. Defining a Hodgkin lymphoma population for novel therapeutics after relapse from autologous hematopoietic cell transplant. Leuk Lymphoma 2013;54(11):2531–3.
26. Martin A, Fernandez-Jimenez MC, Caballero MD, et al. Long-term follow-up in patients treated with Mini-BEAM as salvage therapy for relapsed or refractory Hodgkin's disease. Br J Haematol 2001;113(1):161–71.
27. Czyz A, Lojko-Dankowska A, Dytfeld D, et al. Prognostic factors and long-term outcome of autologous haematopoietic stem cell transplantation following a uniform-modified BEAM-conditioning regimen for patients with refractory or relapsed Hodgkin lymphoma: a single-center experience. Med Oncol 2013; 30(3):611.
28. Linch DC, Winfield D, Goldstone AH, et al. Dose intensification with autologous bone-marrow transplantation in relapsed and resistant Hodgkin's disease: results of a BNLI randomised trial. Lancet 1993;341(8852):1051–4.

29. Schmitz N, Linch DC, Dreger P, et al. Randomised trial of filgrastim-mobilised peripheral blood progenitor cell transplantation versus autologous bone-marrow transplantation in lymphoma patients. Lancet 1996;347(8998):353–7.
30. Schmitz N, Pfistner B, Sextro M, et al. Aggressive conventional chemotherapy compared with high-dose chemotherapy with autologous haemopoietic stem-cell transplantation for relapsed chemosensitive Hodgkin's disease: a randomised trial. Lancet 2002;359(9323):2065–71.
31. Aparicio J, Segura A, Garcera S, et al. ESHAP is an active regimen for relapsing Hodgkin's disease. Ann Oncol 1999;10(5):593–5.
32. Fernandez de Larrea C, Martinez C, Gaya A, et al. Salvage chemotherapy with alternating MINE-ESHAP regimen in relapsed or refractory Hodgkin's lymphoma followed by autologous stem-cell transplantation. Ann Oncol 2010;21(6): 1211–6.
33. Rodriguez J, Rodriguez MA, Fayad L, et al. ASHAP: a regimen for cytoreduction of refractory or recurrent Hodgkin's disease. Blood 1999;93(11):3632–6.
34. Josting A, Rudolph C, Reiser M, et al. Time-intensified dexamethasone/cisplatin/cytarabine: an effective salvage therapy with low toxicity in patients with relapsed and refractory Hodgkin's disease. Ann Oncol 2002;13(10):1628–35.
35. Baetz T, Belch A, Couban S, et al. Gemcitabine, dexamethasone and cisplatin is an active and non-toxic chemotherapy regimen in relapsed or refractory Hodgkin's disease: a phase II study by the National Cancer Institute of Canada Clinical Trials Group. Ann Oncol 2003;14(12):1762–7.
36. Bartlett NL, Niedzwiecki D, Johnson JL, et al. Gemcitabine, vinorelbine, and pegylated liposomal doxorubicin (GVD), a salvage regimen in relapsed Hodgkin's lymphoma: CALGB 59804. Ann Oncol 2007;18(6):1071–9.
37. Santoro A, Magagnoli M, Spina M, et al. Ifosfamide, gemcitabine, and vinorelbine: a new induction regimen for refractory and relapsed Hodgkin's lymphoma. Haematologica 2007;92(1):35–41.
38. Bishton MJ, Lush RJ, Byrne JL, et al. Ifosphamide, etoposide and epirubicin is an effective combined salvage and peripheral blood stem cell mobilisation regimen for transplant-eligible patients with non-Hodgkin lymphoma and Hodgkin disease. Br J Haematol 2007;136(5):752–61.
39. Shafey M, Duan Q, Russell J, et al. Double high-dose therapy with dose-intensive cyclophosphamide, etoposide, cisplatin (DICEP) followed by high-dose melphalan and autologous stem cell transplantation for relapsed/refractory Hodgkin lymphoma. Leuk Lymphoma 2012;53(4):596–602.
40. Sibon D, Ertault M, Al Nawakil C, et al. Combined ifosfamide, etoposide and ox-alipatin chemotherapy, a low-toxicity regimen for first-relapsed or refractory Hodgkin lymphoma after ABVD/EBVP: a prospective monocentre study on 34 patients. Br J Haematol 2011;153(2):191–8.
41. Martinez C, Rodriguez-Calvillo M, Terol MJ, et al. Salvage treatment with ofatumumab and ESHAP (O-ESHAP) for patients with relapsed or refractory classical hodgkin's lymphoma after first-line chemotherapy: interim analysis of a Phase II Trial of the Spanish Group of Lymphoma and Bone Marrow Transplantation (GELTAMO). Blood (ASH Annual Meeting Abstracts) 2012;120(21):1630.
42. Proctor SJ, Jackson GH, Lennard A, et al. Strategic approach to the management of Hodgkin's disease incorporating salvage therapy with high-dose ifosfamide, etoposide and epirubicin: a Northern Region Lymphoma Group study (UK). Ann Oncol 2003;14(Suppl 1):i47–50.
43. Sasse S, Alram M, Mueller H, et al. Prognostic relevance of dose-density of DHAP-reinduction therapy in relapsed HL: an analysis of the German

Hodgkin-Study Group (GHSG). Blood (ASH Annual Meeting Abstracts) 2012; 120(21):552.

44. Rancea M, Monsef I, von Tresckow B, et al. High-dose chemotherapy followed by autologous stem cell transplantation for patients with relapsed/refractory Hodgkin lymphoma. Cochrane Database Syst Rev 2013;(6):CD009411.

45. Lane AA, McAfee SL, Kennedy J, et al. High-dose chemotherapy with busulfan and cyclophosphamide and autologous stem cell rescue in patients with Hodgkin lymphoma. Leuk Lymphoma 2011;52(7):1363–6.

46. Santos EC, Sessions J, Hutcherson D, et al. Long-term outcome of Hodgkin disease patients following high-dose busulfan, etoposide, cyclophosphamide, and autologous stem cell transplantation–a similar experience. Biol Blood Marrow Transplant 2007;13(6):746–7.

47. Di Ianni M, Ballanti S, Iodice G, et al. High-dose thiotepa, etoposide and carboplatin as conditioning regimen for autologous stem cell transplantation in patients with high-risk Hodgkin's lymphoma. Hematology 2012;17(1):23–7.

48. Ganguly S, Jain V, Divine C, et al. BU, melphalan and thiotepa as a preparative regimen for auto-transplantation in Hodgkin's disease. Bone Marrow Transplant 2012;47(2):311–2.

49. Kebriaei P, Madden T, Kazerooni R, et al. Intravenous busulfan plus melphalan is a highly effective, well-tolerated preparative regimen for autologous stem cell transplantation in patients with advanced lymphoid malignancies. Biol Blood Marrow Transplant 2011;17(3):412–20.

50. William BM, Loberiza FR Jr, Whalen V, et al. Impact of conditioning regimen on outcome of 2-year disease-free survivors of autologous stem cell transplantation for Hodgkin lymphoma. Clin Lymphoma Myeloma Leuk 2013;13(4):417–23.

51. Nieto Y, Popat U, Anderlini P, et al. Autologous stem cell transplantation for refractory or poor-risk relapsed Hodgkin's lymphoma: effect of the specific high-dose chemotherapy regimen on outcome. Biol Blood Marrow Transplant 2013; 19(3):410–7.

52. Bains T, Chen AI, Lemieux A, et al. Improved outcome with busulfan, melphalan and thiotepa conditioning in autologous hematopoietic stem cell transplant for relapsed/refractory Hodgkin lymphoma. Leuk Lymphoma 2013. [Epub ahead of print].

53. Moskowitz AJ, Yahalom J, Kewalramani T, et al. Pretransplantation functional imaging predicts outcome following autologous stem cell transplantation for relapsed and refractory Hodgkin lymphoma. Blood 2010;116(23):4934–7.

54. Moskowitz CH, Yahalom J, Zelenetz AD, et al. High-dose chemo-radiotherapy for relapsed or refractory Hodgkin lymphoma and the significance of pretransplant functional imaging. Br J Haematol 2010;148(6):890–7.

55. Jabbour E, Hosing C, Ayers G, et al. Pretransplant positive positron emission tomography/gallium scans predict poor outcome in patients with recurrent/refractory Hodgkin lymphoma. Cancer 2007;109(12):2481–9.

56. Smeltzer JP, Cashen AF, Zhang Q, et al. Prognostic significance of FDG-PET in relapsed or refractory classical Hodgkin lymphoma treated with standard salvage chemotherapy and autologous stem cell transplantation. Biol Blood Marrow Transplant 2011;17(11):1646–52.

57. Sucak GT, Ozkurt ZN, Suyani E, et al. Early post-transplantation positron emission tomography in patients with Hodgkin lymphoma is an independent prognostic factor with an impact on overall survival. Ann Hematol 2011;90(11):1329–36.

58. Devillier R, Coso D, Castagna L, et al. Positron emission tomography response at the time of autologous stem cell transplantation predicts outcome of patients

with relapsed and/or refractory Hodgkin's lymphoma responding to prior salvage therapy. Haematologica 2012;97(7):1073–9.

59. Bramanti S, Castagna L, Viviani S, et al. Early response by 18F-fluorodeoxyglucose positron emission tomography (FDG-PET) during salvage chemotherapy in relapsed/refractory Hodgkin's lymphoma (HL) patients could predict the outcome after high dose chemotherapy (HDC). Haematologica 2013;98(S1):S422.

60. Nassi L, Puccini B, Franceschetti S, et al. Role of pre-transplantation positron emission tomography in patients with Hodgkin's lymphoma undergoing autologous stem cell transplant. Haematologica 2013;98(1):S428.

61. Mocikova H, Pytlik R, Markova J, et al. Pre-transplant positron emission tomography in patients with relapsed Hodgkin lymphoma. Leuk Lymphoma 2011; 52(9):1668–74.

62. Moskowitz CH, Matasar MJ, Zelenetz AD, et al. Normalization of pre-ASCT, FDG-PET imaging with second-line, non-cross-resistant, chemotherapy programs improves event-free survival in patients with Hodgkin lymphoma. Blood 2012;119(7):1665–70.

63. Akhtar S, Al-Sugair AS, Abouzied M, et al. Pre-transplant FDG-PET-based survival model in relapsed and refractory Hodgkin's lymphoma: outcome after high-dose chemotherapy and auto-SCT. Bone Marrow Transplant 2013. [Epub ahead of print].

64. Thomson KJ, Kayani I, Ardeshna K, et al. A response-adjusted PET-based transplantation strategy in primary resistant and relapsed Hodgkin Lymphoma. Leukemia 2013;27(6):1419–22.

65. Brice P, Divine M, Simon D, et al. Feasibility of tandem autologous stem-cell transplantation (ASCT) in induction failure or very unfavorable (UF) relapse from Hodgkin's disease (HD). SFGM/GELA Study Group. Ann Oncol 1999; 10(12):1485–8.

66. Castagna L, Magagnoli M, Balzarotti M, et al. Tandem high-dose chemotherapy and autologous stem cell transplantation in refractory/relapsed Hodgkin's lymphoma: a monocenter prospective study. Am J Hematol 2007;82(2):122–7.

67. Fung HC, Stiff P, Schriber J, et al. Tandem autologous stem cell transplantation for patients with primary refractory or poor risk recurrent Hodgkin lymphoma. Biol Blood Marrow Transplant 2007;13(5):594–600.

68. Morschhauser F, Brice P, Ferme C, et al. Risk-adapted salvage treatment with single or tandem autologous stem-cell transplantation for first relapse/refractory Hodgkin's lymphoma: results of the prospective multicenter H96 trial by the GELA/SFGM study group. J Clin Oncol 2008;26(36):5980–7.

69. Dean RM, Kalaycio M, Pohlman B, et al. Tandem Autologous Hematopoietic Progenitor Cell Transplantation (AHPCT) for high-risk hodgkin lymphoma: mature results of a prospective trial. Blood (ASH Annual Meeting Abstracts) 2012; 120(21):1990.

70. Sibon DR, Morschauer M, Ferme F, et al. Long-term outcome of adults with first relapse or refractory Hodgkin Lymphoma treated in the prospective LYSA/SFGM-TC H96 trial. (2013), oral presentations. Hematol Oncol 2013;31: 96–150. http://dx.doi.org/10.1002/hon.2057.

71. Goyal SD, Bartlett NL. Where does brentuximab vedotin fit into the management of patients with Hodgkin lymphoma? Curr Hematol Malig Rep 2012; 7(3):179–85.

72. Moskowitz AJ, Perales MA, Kewalramani T, et al. Outcomes for patients who fail high dose chemoradiotherapy and autologous stem cell rescue for relapsed and primary refractory Hodgkin lymphoma. Br J Haematol 2009;146(2):158–63.

73. Corazzelli G, Angrilli F, D'Arco A, et al. Efficacy and safety of bendamustine for the treatment of patients with recurring Hodgkin lymphoma. Br J Haematol 2013; 160(2):207–15.
74. Younes A, Sureda A, Ben-Yehuda D, et al. Panobinostat in patients with relapsed/refractory Hodgkin's lymphoma after autologous stem-cell transplantation: results of a phase II study. J Clin Oncol 2012;30(18):2197–203.
75. Rothe A, Sasse S, Goergen H, et al. Brentuximab vedotin for relapsed or refractory CD30+ hematologic malignancies: the German Hodgkin Study Group experience. Blood 2012;120(7):1470–2.
76. Gajewski JL, Phillips GL, Sobocinski KA, et al. Bone marrow transplants from HLA-identical siblings in advanced Hodgkin's disease. J Clin Oncol 1996; 14(2):572–8.
77. Milpied N, Fielding AK, Pearce RM, et al. Allogeneic bone marrow transplant is not better than autologous transplant for patients with relapsed Hodgkin's disease. European Group for Blood and Bone Marrow Transplantation. J Clin Oncol 1996;14(4):1291–6.
78. Jones RJ, Piantadosi S, Mann RB, et al. High-dose cytotoxic therapy and bone marrow transplantation for relapsed Hodgkin's disease. J Clin Oncol 1990;8(3): 527–37.
79. Peniket AJ, Ruiz de Elvira MC, Taghipour G, et al. An EBMT registry matched study of allogeneic stem cell transplants for lymphoma: allogeneic transplantation is associated with a lower relapse rate but a higher procedure-related mortality rate than autologous transplantation. Bone Marrow Transplant 2003;31(8): 667–78.
80. Anderson JE, Litzow MR, Appelbaum FR, et al. Allogeneic, syngeneic, and autologous marrow transplantation for Hodgkin's disease: the 21-year Seattle experience. J Clin Oncol 1993;11(12):2342–50.
81. Akpek G, Ambinder RF, Piantadosi S, et al. Long-term results of blood and marrow transplantation for Hodgkin's lymphoma. J Clin Oncol 2001;19(23): 4314–21.
82. Sureda A, Robinson S, Canals C, et al. Reduced-intensity conditioning compared with conventional allogeneic stem-cell transplantation in relapsed or refractory Hodgkin's lymphoma: an analysis from the Lymphoma Working Party of the European Group for Blood and Marrow Transplantation. J Clin Oncol 2008;26(3):455–62.
83. Robinson SP, Goldstone AH, Mackinnon S, et al. Chemoresistant or aggressive lymphoma predicts for a poor outcome following reduced-intensity allogeneic progenitor cell transplantation: an analysis from the Lymphoma Working Party of the European Group for Blood and Bone Marrow Transplantation. Blood 2002;100(13):4310–6.
84. Alvarez I, Sureda A, Caballero MD, et al. Nonmyeloablative stem cell transplantation is an effective therapy for refractory or relapsed Hodgkin lymphoma: results of a Spanish prospective cooperative protocol. Biol Blood Marrow Transplant 2006;12(2):172–83.
85. Peggs KS, Hunter A, Chopra R, et al. Clinical evidence of a graft-versus-Hodgkin's-lymphoma effect after reduced-intensity allogeneic transplantation. Lancet 2005;365(9475):1934–41.
86. Baron F, Storb R, Storer BE, et al. Factors associated with outcomes in allogeneic hematopoietic cell transplantation with nonmyeloablative conditioning after failed myeloablative hematopoietic cell transplantation. J Clin Oncol 2006; 24(25):4150–7.

87. Majhail NS, Weisdorf DJ, Wagner JE, et al. Comparable results of umbilical cord blood and HLA-matched sibling donor hematopoietic stem cell transplantation after reduced-intensity preparative regimen for advanced Hodgkin lymphoma. Blood 2006;107(9):3804–7.
88. Peggs KS, Sureda A, Qian W, et al. Reduced-intensity conditioning for allogeneic haematopoietic stem cell transplantation in relapsed and refractory Hodgkin lymphoma: impact of alemtuzumab and donor lymphocyte infusions on long-term outcomes. Br J Haematol 2007;139(1):70–80.
89. Anderlini P, Saliba R, Acholonu S, et al. Reduced-intensity allogeneic stem cell transplantation in relapsed and refractory Hodgkin's disease: low transplant-related mortality and impact of intensity of conditioning regimen. Bone Marrow Transplant 2005;35(10):943–51.
90. Anderlini P, Saliba R, Acholonu S, et al. Fludarabine-melphalan as a preparative regimen for reduced-intensity conditioning allogeneic stem cell transplantation in relapsed and refractory Hodgkin's lymphoma: the updated M.D. Anderson Cancer Center experience. Haematologica 2008;93(2):257–64.
91. Armand P, Kim HT, Ho VT, et al. Allogeneic transplantation with reduced-intensity conditioning for Hodgkin and non-Hodgkin lymphoma: importance of histology for outcome. Biol Blood Marrow Transplant 2008;14(4):418–25.
92. Burroughs LM, O'Donnell PV, Sandmaier BM, et al. Comparison of outcomes of HLA-matched related, unrelated, or HLA-haploidentical related hematopoietic cell transplantation following nonmyeloablative conditioning for relapsed or re-fractory Hodgkin lymphoma. Biol Blood Marrow Transplant 2008;14(11): 1279–87.
93. Thomson KJ, Peggs KS, Smith P, et al. Superiority of reduced-intensity allogeneic transplantation over conventional treatment for relapse of Hodgkin's lymphoma following autologous stem cell transplantation. Bone Marrow Transplant 2008; 41(9):765–70.
94. Castagna L, Sarina B, Todisco E, et al. Allogeneic stem cell transplantation compared with chemotherapy for poor-risk Hodgkin lymphoma. Biol Blood Marrow Transplant 2009;15(4):432–8.
95. Devetten MP, Hari PN, Carreras J, et al. Unrelated donor reduced-intensity allo-geneic hematopoietic stem cell transplantation for relapsed and refractory Hodgkin lymphoma. Biol Blood Marrow Transplant 2009;15(1):109–17.
96. Robinson SP, Sureda A, Canals C, et al. Reduced intensity conditioning alloge-neic stem cell transplantation for Hodgkin's lymphoma: identification of prog-nostic factors predicting outcome. Haematologica 2009;94(2):230–8.
97. Kuruvilla J, Pintilie M, Stewart D, et al. Outcomes of reduced-intensity condition-ing allo-SCT for Hodgkin's lymphoma: a national review by the Canadian Blood and Marrow Transplant Group. Bone Marrow Transplant 2010;45(7):1253–5.
98. Sarina B, Castagna L, Farina L, et al. Allogeneic transplantation improves the overall and progression-free survival of Hodgkin lymphoma patients relapsing after autologous transplantation: a retrospective study based on the time of HLA typing and donor availability. Blood 2010;115(18):3671–7.
99. Chen R, Palmer JM, Popplewell L, et al. Reduced intensity allogeneic hemato-poietic cell transplantation can induce durable remission in heavily pretreated relapsed Hodgkin lymphoma. Ann Hematol 2011;90(7):803–8.
100. Johansson JE, Remberger M, Lazarevic V, et al. Allogeneic haematopoietic stem-cell transplantation with reduced intensity conditioning for advanced stage Hodgkin's lymphoma in Sweden: high incidence of post transplant lymphopro-liferative disorder. Bone Marrow Transplant 2011;46(6):870–5.

101. Anderlini P, Saliba RM, Ledesma C, et al. Gemcitabine, fludarabine and melphalan as a reduced-intensity conditioning regimen for allogeneic stem cell transplant in relapsed and refractory Hodgkin lymphoma: preliminary results. Leuk Lymphoma 2012;53(3):499–502.
102. Sobol U, Rodriguez T, Smith S, et al. Long term follow-up of allogeneic transplantation using BEAM chemotherapy for patients with Hodgkin's Lymphoma who relapse after autologous transplantation: importance of minimal residual disease at transplant. Blood (ASH Annual Meeting Abstracts) 2012;120(21):3131.
103. Sureda A, Canals C, Arranz R, et al. Allogeneic stem cell transplantation after reduced intensity conditioning in patients with relapsed or refractory Hodgkin's lymphoma. Results of the HDR-ALLO study - a prospective clinical trial by the Grupo Espanol de Linfomas/Trasplante de Medula Osea (GEL/TAMO) and the Lymphoma Working Party of the European Group for Blood and Marrow Transplantation. Haematologica 2012;97(2):310–7.
104. Chen R, Forman S, Palmer J, et al. Two-year follow-up of patients with relapsed/refractory Hodgkin treated with Brentuximab Vedotin prior to reduced intensity allogeneic hematopoietic cell transplantation. Hematol Oncol 2013;31(Suppl 1): 96–150.
105. Chen R, Palmer JM, Thomas SH, et al. Brentuximab vedotin enables successful reduced-intensity allogeneic hematopoietic cell transplantation in patients with relapsed or refractory Hodgkin lymphoma. Blood 2012;119(26):6379–81.
106. Marcais A, Porcher R, Robin M, et al. Disease status and stem cell source impact on the results of reduced intensity conditioning transplant for Hodgkin lymphoma: a retrospective study from the French Society of Bone Marrow Graft Transplantation and Cellular Therapy. Haematologica 2013;98(9): 1467–75.
107. Bacigalupo A, Castagna L, Raiola A, et al. Unmanipulated haploidentical bone marrow transplantation following non-myeloablative conditioning and post-transplant cyclophosphamide for advanced Hodgkin's lymphoma. Haematologica 2013;98(S1):67.
108. Anderlini P, Champlin RE. Reduced intensity conditioning for allogeneic stem cell transplantation in relapsed and refractory Hodgkin lymphoma: where do we stand? Biol Blood Marrow Transplant 2006;12(6):599–602.
109. Todisco E, Castagna L, Sarina B, et al. Reduced-intensity allogeneic transplantation in patients with refractory or progressive Hodgkin's disease after high-dose chemotherapy and autologous stem cell infusion. Eur J Haematol 2007;78(4): 322–9.
110. Dodero A, Crocchiolo R, Patriarca F, et al. Pretransplantation [18-F] fluorodeoxyglucose positron emission tomography scan predicts outcome in patients with recurrent Hodgkin lymphoma or aggressive non-Hodgkin lymphoma undergoing reduced-intensity conditioning followed by allogeneic stem cell transplantation. Cancer 2010;116(21):5001–11.
111. Corradini P, Sarina B, Farina L. Allogeneic transplantation for Hodgkin's lymphoma. Br J Haematol 2011;152(3):261–72.
112. Messer M, Steinzen A, Vervolgyi E, et al. Unrelated and alternative donor allogeneic stem cell transplant in patients with relapsed or refractory Hodgkin lymphoma: a systematic review. Leuk Lymphoma 2013. [Epub ahead of print].
113. Peggs KS, Kayani I, Edwards N, et al. Donor lymphocyte infusions modulate relapse risk in mixed chimeras and induce durable salvage in relapsed patients after T-cell-depleted allogeneic transplantation for Hodgkin's lymphoma. J Clin Oncol 2011;29(8):971–8.

114. Anderlini P, Saliba R, Acholonu S, et al. Donor leukocyte infusions in recurrent Hodgkin lymphoma following allogeneic stem cell transplant: 10-year experience at the M. D. Anderson Cancer Center. Leuk Lymphoma 2012;53(6): 1239–41.

115. Anderlini P, Acholonu SA, Okoroji GJ, et al. Donor leukocyte infusions in relapsed Hodgkin's lymphoma following allogeneic stem cell transplantation: CD3+ cell dose, GVHD and disease response. Bone Marrow Transplant 2004;34(6):511–4.

116. Greaves PJ, Gribben JG. Demonstration of durable graft versus lymphoma effects in Hodgkin's lymphoma. J Clin Oncol 2011;29(8):952–3.

117. Furst S, Bouabdallah R, Coso D, et al. High response rate and no treatment related mortality after brentuximab vedotin salvage therapy followed by reduced intensity conditioning regimen allogeneic stem cell transplantation (RIC-ALLO) in patients with CD 30+ lymphomas. ASH Annual Meeting Abstracts 2012; 120(21):4526.

118. Wannesson L, Bargetzi M, Cairoli A, et al. Autotransplant for Hodgkin lymphoma after failure of upfront BEACOPP escalated (bleomycin, etoposide, doxorubicin, cyclophosphamide, vincristine, procarbazine and prednisone). Leuk Lymphoma 2013;54(1):36–40.

119. Gopal AK, Ramchandren R, O'Connor OA, et al. Safety and efficacy of brentuximab vedotin for Hodgkin lymphoma recurring after allogeneic stem cell transplantation. Blood 2012;120(3):560–8.

120. Theurich S, Malcher J, Wennhold K, et al. Brentuximab vedotin combined with donor lymphocyte infusions for early relapse of Hodgkin lymphoma after allogeneic stem-cell transplantation induces tumor-specific immunity and sustained clinical remission. J Clin Oncol 2013;31(5):e59–63.

Index

Note: Page numbers of article titles are in **boldface** type.

Hematol Oncol Clin N Am 28 (2014) 149–154
http://dx.doi.org/10.1016/S0889-8588(13)00175-5
0889-8588/14/$ – see front matter © 2014 Elsevier Inc. All rights reserved.

Printed and bound by CPI Group (UK) Ltd, Croydon, CR0 4YY

03/10/2024

01040478-0015